Surviving, Existing, or Living

For professionals working with people who experience severe psychosis, increasing empirical evidence for the benefits of psychotherapy for psychosis has been especially welcome. Given the limitations of medication-only approaches and the need for an expanded perspective, including for those diagnosed with schizophrenia, *Surviving, Existing, or Living* takes a fresh look at severe psychosis, offering a heuristic model for understanding psychosis along a continuum of severity, from the extreme experience of acutely impairing psychosis to a more enriched life experience.

Pamela R. Fuller emphasizes that facilitating recovery from psychosis requires appropriately and effectively matching the type and timing of interventions to client readiness and capabilities. The need to consider each individual according to which of three primary issues/phases preoccupy the person with psychosis is essential for tailoring treatment. She identifies these phases as:

- Surviving Phase – preoccupation with survival
- Existing Phase – preoccupation with restriction of life experiences in order to cope
- Living Phase – preoccupation with quality of life and relationships.

Surviving, Existing, or Living examines the rationale for these three phases, and provides details of phase-specific treatment interventions as well as a "how to" guide for facilitating engagement and for determining "what to do when," including with those experiencing acute, severe psychosis. Rich clinical case examples are provided to highlight concepts and the types of interventions. Trauma-specific and group interventions for psychosis are also described, as well as ways to foster resilience in the professional who works with individuals with psychosis.

Surviving, Existing, or Living offers a detailed guide to help individuals experiencing psychosis move from suffering to recovery, beyond surviving or existing toward more fully living. The book will be essential reading for professionals in the fields of psychology; psychiatry; counseling; medicine; social work; nursing; occupational, recreational, and vocational therapies; experience-based experts; and students.

Pamela R. Fuller is a clinical psychologist with extensive experience working across the continuum of care with children, adolescents, and adults who have severe psychological problems. She is currently in private practice in Evanston, Wyoming, USA.

The International Society for Psychological and Social Approaches to Psychosis Book Series

Series editors: Brian Martindale and Alison Summers

ISPS (The International Society for Psychological and Social Approaches to Psychosis) has a history stretching back more than fifty years during which it has witnessed the relentless pursuit of biological explanations for psychosis. The tide has been turning in recent years and there is a welcome international resurgence of interest in a range of psychological factors that have considerable explanatory power and therapeutic possibilities. Governments, professional groups, people with personal experience of psychosis and family members are increasingly expecting interventions that involve more talking and listening. Many now regard practitioners skilled in psychological therapies as an essential component of the care of people with psychosis.

ISPS is a global society. It aims to promote psychological and social approaches both to understanding and to treating psychosis. It also aims to bring together different perspectives on these issues. ISPS is composed of individuals, networks and institutional members from a wide range of backgrounds and is especially concerned that those with personal experience of psychosis and their family members are fully involved in our activities alongside practitioners and researchers, and that all benefit from this. Our members recognize the potential humanitarian and therapeutic potential of skilled psychological understanding and therapy in the field of psychosis and ISPS embraces a wide spectrum of approaches from psychodynamic, systemic, cognitive, and arts therapies to the need-adapted approaches, family and group therapies and residential therapeutic communities.

We are also most interested in establishing meaningful dialogue with those practitioners and researchers who are more familiar with biological-based approaches. There is increasing empirical evidence for the interaction of genes and biology with the emotional and social environment, and there are important examples of such interactions in the fields of trauma, attachment relationships in the family and in social settings and with professionals.

ISPS activities include regular international and national conferences, newsletters and email discussion groups. Routledge has recognized the importance of our field in publishing both the book series and the ISPS journal: *Psychosis: Psychological, Social and Integrative Approaches,* with the two complementing one another. The book series started in 2004 and by 2012 had thirteen volumes with several more in preparation.

A wide range of topics are covered and we hope this reflects some success in our aim of bringing together a rich range of perspectives.

The book series is intended as a resource for a broad range of mental health professionals as well as those developing and implementing policy and people whose interest in psychosis is at a personal level. We aim for rigorous academic standards and at the same time accessibility to a wide range of readers, and for the books to promote the ideas of clinicians and researchers who may be well known in some countries but not so familiar in others. Our overall intention is to encourage the dissemination of existing knowledge and ideas, promote productive debate, and encourage more research in a most important field whose secrets certainly do not all reside in the neurosciences.

For more information about ISPS, email isps@isps.org or visit our website, www.isps.org.

For more information about the journal *Psychosis* visit www.isps.org/index.php/publications/journal

Models of Madness: Psychological, Social and Biological Approaches to Schizophrenia
Edited by John Read, Loren R. Mosher and Richard P. Bentall

Psychoses: An Integrative Perspective
Edited by Johan Cullberg

Evolving Psychosis: Different Stages, Different Treatments
Edited by Jan Olav Johanessen, Brian V. Martindale and Johan Cullberg

Family and Multi-Family Work with Psychosis
Gerd-Ragna Block Thorsen, Trond Gronnestad and Anne Lise Oxenvad

Experiences of Mental Health In-Patient Care: Narratives from Service Users, Carers and Professionals
Edited by Mark Hardcastle, David Kennard, Sheila Grandison and Leonard Fagin

Psychotherapies for the Psychoses: Theoretical, Cultural, and Clinical Integration
Edited by John Gleeson, Eión Killackey and Helen Krstev

Therapeutic Communities for Psychosis: Philosophy, History and Clinical Practice
Edited by John Gale, Alba Realpe and Enrico Pedriali

Beyond Medication: Therapeutic Engagement and the Recovery from Psychosis
Edited by David Garfield and Daniel Mackler

Making Sense of Madness: Contesting the Meaning of Schizophrenia
Jim Geekie and John Read

Psychotherapeutic Approaches to Schizophrenia Psychosis
Edited by Yrjö O. Alanen, Manuel González de Chávez, Ann-Louise S. Silver and Brian Martindale

CBT for Psychosis: A Symptom-based Approach
Edited by Roger Hagen, Douglas Turkington, Torkil Berge and Rolf W. Gråwe

Psychosis as a Personal Crisis: An Experience-based Approach
Edited by Marius Romme and Sandra Escher

Psychosis and Emotion: The Role of Emotions in Understanding Psychosis, Therapy and Recovery
Edited by Andrew Gumley, Alf Gillham, Kathy Taylor and Matthias Schwannauer

Experiencing Psychosis: Personal and Professional Perspectives
Edited by Jim Geekie, Patte Randal, Debra Lampshire and John Read

Insanity and Divinity: Studies in Psychosis and Spirituality
Edited by John Gale, Michael Robson and Georgia Rapsomatioti

Surviving, Existing, or Living: Phase-specific Therapy for Severe Psychosis
Pamela R. Fuller

Surviving, Existing, or Living

Phase-specific therapy for severe psychosis

Pamela R. Fuller

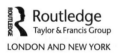

Routledge
Taylor & Francis Group

LONDON AND NEW YORK

First published 2013
by Routledge
27 Church Road, Hove, East Sussex BN3 2FA

Simultaneously published in the USA and Canada
by Routledge
711 Third Avenue, New York, NY 10017

Routledge is an imprint of the Taylor and Francis Group, an informa business

British Library Cataloguing in Publication Data
A catalogue record for this book is available from the British Library

Library of Congress Cataloging in Publication Data
Fuller, Pamela R.
  Surviving, existing, or living : phase-specific therapy for severe
  psychosis / Pamela R. Fuller.
     pages cm
  Includes bibliographical references.
  1. Psychoses – Treatment. 2. Psychotherapy. I. Title.
  RC512.F85 2013
  616.89'14–dc23   2012049530

ISBN: 978-0-415-51661-7 (hbk)
ISBN: 978-0-415-51662-4 (pbk)
ISBN: 978-0-203-77744-2 (ebk)

Typeset in Garamond
by HWA Text and Data Management, London

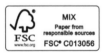

Printed and bound in Great Britain by
TJ International Ltd, Padstow, Cornwall

Contents

Acknowledgements

I am very grateful to the many people who have helped to make this book possible. First, to the many individuals with severe psychosis who have let me know them and allowed me to walk with them as they worked to regain a greater sense of themselves and satisfaction in their lives. I have been changed by my experiences with them.

To Brian Martindale and Alison Summers, the editors of the ISPS series, for their wisdom, insight, and guidance in writing this book.

To Perry, for being the first to encourage me to publish. To Adam, who steadfastly supported me in this endeavor and provided extensive, insightful edits. To Benjamin and Breila and extended family for their support, and to the many colleagues across disciplines who have contributed to these ideas.

Introduction

"I don't want voices anymore, but I can't survive without them."

These are exciting times in the expansion of our understanding and treatment of psychosis. We are progressing from a view of psychosis as a solely biological condition to a biopsychosocial perspective, which recognizes that complex factors contribute to the etiology and manifestations of the diverse forms of psychosis. In particular, there is increasing understanding that experiences of psychosis can range from more severe forms (characterized by an extreme disturbance in the sense of self, highly interfering and/or distressing hallucinations or delusions, and significant impairment in functioning) to the less interfering experiences of a higher functioning individual who hears voices or maintains a circumscribed delusion. This reflects a radical and necessary shift from an oversimplified bifurcation of "psychotic" or "not psychotic" to one that considers the intensity and severity of interference of psychosis in an individual's life.

Our broadening to a dimensional perspective of psychosis has been accompanied by advances in treatment as well. As part of this progress, there is strong, accumulating evidence for the role of psychological therapies in the treatment of the psychoses, including for those diagnosed with schizophrenia. Cognitive-behavioral therapies, psychodynamic therapies, self-psychology approaches, family therapies, mindfulness techniques, multidisciplinary, psychosocial programs, and other approaches each are contributing diverse, important practices for enhancing treatment efficacy. These approaches target improving treatment outcome, including enhancing a sense of self and interpersonal experiences, increasing adaptive, reality-based coping, reducing distress and intrusion of hallucinations and delusions, and improving overall functioning.

These contemporary approaches reflect dramatic and much needed progress away from a medication-only approach to psychosis. Treatment with antipsychotic medication alone has been shown to be insufficient and to be associated with severe side effects, such as diabetes mellitus, hyperlipidemia, and obesity. There also are poor compliance rates with antipsychotic medications and negative symptoms, social skill deficits, depression, and cognitive difficulties often persist. Further, relapse rates for medication-alone approaches remain high, even when medication adherence is monitored. These limitations of medication-only, illness-model approaches have prompted development of more comprehensive recovery models, which include a renewed focus on psychological interventions for psychosis.

By creating a means for determining which interventions to conduct when, many of the diverse treatment approaches currently in use may be integrated into a comprehensive, strategic approach to psychosis. In response, this book offers a conceptual framework, the Surviving, Existing, or Living (SEL) model, as a method for assessing the person's often fluctuating psychological capabilities and needs and choosing the type and timing of interventions accordingly. As such, the model allows for integration of the many therapies in use (including but not limited to cognitive-behavioral therapies, psychodynamically informed approaches, and family therapies) into a strategic approach to care and recovery that strives to enhance alignment between therapeutic interventions and the individual's psychological state and psychological readiness. The model conceptualizes psychosis along a continuum of severity, based on such factors as the extent of self-definition, interpersonal awareness, distressing hallucinations, or delusions, and awareness of thoughts and emotions. Three general phases (Surviving, Existing, and Living) of the model fall along the continuum, reflecting different levels of severity. The specificity of the features described for each phase allows for characterizing the immediate psychological state of the person to guide effective pacing of therapeutic interventions. In addition, the treatment approach can be quickly modified in response to the rapid changes in psychological status that can occur. This suggested approach to treatment planning is in keeping with contemporary clinical and empirical literature which, instead of advocating for a single treatment approach to psychosis, indicates that certain treatment interventions may be more effective at particular times, depending on the individual's status.

Surviving, Existing, or Living also presents a specific "how-to" guide for providing psychological services for the most severe forms of psychosis, including for those with a diagnosis of schizophrenia, across the different phases. The most severe form of psychosis refers to those who, at some point, have experienced a complete loss of awareness of existence of the self (and the accompanying significant disturbances in thinking, behavior, affect, and perception) during an acute episode. Such an episode falls at the furthest, most extreme, endpoint on the dimensional scale of psychotic experience, and includes many diagnosed with schizophrenia. Phase-specific treatment strategies designed to foster and maintain engagement and facilitate progression from the Surviving to the Existing and Living Phases are described, with the use of illustrative case examples. Because there has been less attention to those in an acute or chronically acute phase, special attention is given to detailed descriptions of interventions for the Surviving Phase (i.e., acute, severe psychosis). In addition, parallels between phase-specific treatment for psychosis and current trauma treatment models are highlighted, to expand the mental health professional's understanding of how maltreatment may contribute to psychosis. Methods for effective, trauma-informed intervention are also described, as well as applications of the SEL model to group therapies. Finally, the importance of fortifying the mental health professional who works with individuals with severe psychoses is explored.

Engagement and treatment can be especially challenging with those who have experienced more severe, chronic forms of psychosis and have been treated within a medical model, particularly in comparison to treatment with those experiencing a first-episode psychosis initially approached from a recovery-oriented perspective. When a psychosis persists over time, removal from reality into hallucinations and delusions can become an automatic, entrenched means of coping with stressors and with people. Years of being ostracized from society and separated from home communities, being told one has a chronic, debilitating brain disease, and living a restricted life, can result in a narrowed identity as a patient or as a disease (i.e., "a schizophrenic"). For such individuals, and for those who work with them, the idea of having a satisfying life can be difficult to imagine. Particularly if the person has been treated within a medical model for years, the shift to the collaborative, hope-instilling perspective of recovery-oriented mental health care can be a much-needed, yet startling, change. The ideas in this book originally were developed to assist mental health professionals in making this shift in approach by describing ways to facilitate engagement and work with such individuals.

While *Surviving, Existing, or Living* places particular emphasis on the most severe forms of psychosis, many aspects of the model are applicable to assessing and treating less debilitating forms of psychosis as well. For example, the model may assist in tailoring the intensive, community-based services that are being provided as early interventions in psychosis, including for first-episode psychosis. Further, although the book has particular emphasis on psychological services for psychosis, the model has relevance for tailoring the treatment planning of various disciplines, including nursing, social work, pharmacy, psychiatry, experience-based experts, and occupational, vocational, and recreational therapists.

The overall purpose of *Surviving, Existing, or Living* is to offer a heuristic model for conceptualizing psychosis dimensionally and for matching interventions to the individual's psychological state. It also offers methods for providing psychological services to persons with the most severe forms of psychosis, including those with a diagnosis of schizophrenia, with the goal of increasing the motivation and skill of mental health professionals who provide services to individuals for whom a relationship is especially difficult, but particularly important. In essence, this book offers a means for helping individuals move from suffering to recovery, beyond surviving toward more fully living.

Chapter 1

The three phases of severe psychosis
Surviving, existing, and living

"My life is artificial."

The above statement, which came from a man who was diagnosed with schizophrenia and had been at a psychiatric hospital in the United States for many years, poignantly expresses what the experience of severe psychosis can be like: a false self and a false life. Can we, as mental health professionals, help someone like this progress from an experience of an "artificial" life to one of more fully living in a real and satisfying way? This book offers a guide on how to do that. The first step toward accomplishing that goal is to understand the most severe form of psychosis (including the diagnostic category of schizophrenia), not as a list of symptoms, but as a complex human experience. This first chapter delineates specific characteristics of the most severe form of psychosis, particularly in relation to past and current descriptions of schizophrenia. This is followed by a description of the Surviving, Existing, or Living (SEL) model as a means to conceptualize this varying, complex, and often fluctuating experience by delineating features along a continuum, which are divided into three general phases of severity. Because selecting and implementing treatment interventions that match the individual's immediate presentation and psychological readiness is a crucial aspect to enhancing treatment effectiveness, the SEL model also offers a method for determining what interventions to use at particular times. An overview of the general types and objectives of interventions for each phase is given in this chapter, with specific details provided in subsequent chapters.

The emphasis in this chapter and throughout the book is on the conceptualization and treatment of the most severe forms of psychosis, for those who – in addition to hallucinations or delusions – experience, at some point, a loss of a sense of self. Throughout this book, reference to those with "severe psychosis" and "the most severe form of psychosis" will pertain to this subset of individuals, which includes many of those diagnosed with schizophrenia, as well as some who have been misdiagnosed or never labeled.

Characteristics of severe psychosis

The problem in defining characteristics of severe psychosis

Although there are extensive concerns and disagreement about the current diagnostic category of schizophrenia, most would likely agree that there is a subset of individuals whose psychosis is far more distressing and impairing, who – in addition to having hallucinations or delusions – exhibit significant problems in thinking and in functioning. Further, psychosis in its most severe form regresses into a terrifying state of existential uncertainty. Some clinicians and researchers, from the remote past as well as the present, consider this to be a defining characteristic of those diagnosed with schizophrenia. Those with other forms of psychosis, as well as some who have been diagnosed with schizophrenia, do not regress to this extreme of questioning their very existence.

Problems with the construct validity of the term "schizophrenia" complicate conceptualization of severe psychosis as well as confound research into etiology and treatment efficacy. It has been recognized since Bleuler (1911/1950) that "schizophrenia" may actually represent a collection of disorders. The number of psychiatric disorders that include psychotic symptoms indicates that there are many variants of psychosis, with different causes, manifestations, and outcomes. Schizophrenia currently is defined by the experience of hallucinations, delusions, disorganized speech, grossly disorganized or catatonic behavior, negative symptoms such as flat affect, alogia, or avolition, thought disturbances (e.g., thought broadcasting, insertion, or withdrawal) and delusions of control (American Psychiatric Association, 2000; World Health Organization, 1994). It is inevitable that these criteria for schizophrenia – and for other, related diagnostic categories – will change as our understanding of psychosis, and its various presentations, advances. In particular, the varying forms and degrees of psychosis necessitate a dimensional perspective rather than discrete categories for psychosis. Understanding the most severe form of psychosis as defined by the complete loss of awareness of existence of the self in the most acute, regressed, phase (and the accompanying severe disturbances in thinking, behavior, affect, and perception) would place such presentations at the furthest, and most severe, endpoint on the dimensional scale of psychotic experience. With this approach, "schizophrenia" is distinguished more by severity, including in self-disturbance, from other, less impairing, psychotic experiences as well as from other mental health problems. The dimensional perspective also facilitates a move away from simplistic notions of being "sick" or "well," "psychotic" or "not psychotic."

Additional characteristics of severe psychosis

In addition to the contemporary diagnostic criteria, the following features have been emphasized in the clinical and empirical literature as distinguishing features of schizophrenia and are proffered here to characterize the subgroup of the most severe form of psychosis.

Disturbance in sense of self

The clinical literature has long described schizophrenia as a fundamental disorder of the self. For example, in 1896, Kraepelin (as cited in Sass and Parnas, 2003) described the "loss of inner unity of consciousness" as a core feature of dementia praecox that was like being "an orchestra without a conductor." Characteristic symptoms of schizophrenia in the *Diagnostic and Statistical Manual*, 3rd edition, revised (DSM-III-R: American Psychiatric Association, 1987) included a disturbance in the sense of self, as evidenced by "extreme perplexity about one's own identity" and the ICD-10 (World Health Organization, 1994) describes a "disturbance of the basic functions that give a normal person a feeling of individuality and uniqueness." Karon and Vandenbos (1981) referred to this central issue as "existential terror." More recently, Sass and Parnas (2003) have described schizophrenia as an "ipseity disturbance," a fundamental disorder of the self characterized by a diminished awareness of one's existence. Lysaker *et al.* (2008) referred to this as "the diminishment of self-experience."

It is not uncommon for this uncertainty about existence and self-diminishment to be directly stated. For example, a man diagnosed with schizophrenia said, "I think I am dead but don't know it yet." Another stated that, "The real Jeanne S. died three years ago. This is the third Jeanne S. and is just a robot." When another client was asked what he looked like, he became quite anxious and said, "I don't know. I don't have a picture of me from when I was a kid." When another was asked what she sees when she looks in the mirror, she replied, "All I see is my voices." For these individuals, in a most regressed state, their fear is that they may not exist. In essence, the fundamental question in this most acute phase is not "Who am I?" but "Am I?" This, then, is a hallmark of the most severe psychoses that differentiates it from other psychotic disorders: at his/her "worst," the person loses the knowledge and reassurance of existence that is generally an implicit, fundamental tenet of the human experience.

With a slightly more developed self-structure (i.e., a better defined sense of self), this threat to existence can manifest as a fear of annihilation, which reflects awareness of existence, but an existence that is precarious. That is, the person exists but is terrified of being killed, such as with persecutory delusions that reflect existential threat. For example, a client who expresses delusional beliefs that the CIA or some other secret or security service is after him reflects, in part, a fear of being killed (as well as some grandiosity that they are important enough for a national secret service to want them killed). Threat to existence can also manifest as fears of falling apart or disintegrating, of being engulfed (Laing, 1960), or as somatic delusions. The sense of the self as a coherent, separate individual develops as the person with severe psychosis reconstitutes. This may be evident in an increased ability to express opinions and ideas and an increased awareness of others and of their surroundings.

Limited awareness of others

Significant impairments in social functioning in those diagnosed with schizophrenia are well-known. The severe social impairment during the acute phase of more severe psychosis is easily understood, given the level of distress and perceived threat, the disruption in the inherent organization of the self, and the focus on internal stimuli. Specifically, when an individual is terrified that s/he does not exist or perceives an extreme threat to existence, the attention is turned inward, perceptions are distorted, and there is little awareness of anything outside the self. As the individual reconstitutes and safety and sense of self increases, there is greater definition between self and other and, concomitantly, increasing awareness of others. However, even as the person stabilizes, problems in social relating may remain, including limited conversational skills, deficits in accurately reading social cues, and limited assertiveness.

Constant sense of threat/high arousal

During an acute psychotic episode, the individual perceives the world as a threatening and unsafe place and readily misperceives experiences as dangerous. This is accompanied by a higher arousal level, physiologically and emotionally. For example, acutely psychotic individuals frequently present as highly agitated, pacing, sleeping less, distracted by distressing voices or beliefs, talking rapidly, and paranoid. It is obvious, at these times, that the individual is highly aroused physiologically and emotionally under the perceived experience of intense threat to personal safety. However, a greater extreme of arousal is evident in the person who presents with severe emotional restriction, numbing, and the feeling of detachment (dissociation) reflective of an extreme stress response to a perceived threat to one's existence; a reaction frequently described in the trauma literature as the "freeze" response (Levine, 1997). This is similar to an animal that plays dead as a final effort to protect itself from being killed (see Karon and Vandenbos, 1981, and their description of catatonia as a survival response to existential terror). The major tranquilizers that have been used to treat acute psychosis and the anti-anxiety medications used as the initial pharmacologic intervention for first-episode psychosis in some countries (Spencer *et al.*, 2001) target this high arousal. An essential aspect of stabilization of the person, then, is both the reduction in perceived threat, and in concomitant emotional and physiological arousal.

Limited awareness of thoughts

An additional characteristic of a person with severe psychosis is a limited awareness of personal thoughts, which is a fundamental aspect of metacognitive abilities. Rudimentary self-structure (i.e., emerging awareness of the self as made up of different, interrelated parts) is necessary to be able to examine personal thoughts and feelings as passing states rather than as an immediate, global self-depiction. That is, a person has to be able to discern that one *has* thoughts and feelings rather than one *is* his or her thoughts or feelings. In addition to the lack of awareness of cognitive processes, there seems to be an inverse relationship between logical thought processes and the degree of psychosis. That is, the more psychotic the individual, the less coherent and logical the content of speech. Increasing problems in logical, coherent thought processes may be manifested in flight of ideas, loosening of associations, or tangentiality. Furthermore, neuropsychological investigations of individuals diagnosed with schizophrenia indicate significant cognitive impairment, including in working memory, processing speed, verbal learning, attention, and executive function, even as acute psychosis abates (Hugdahl and Calhoun, 2010). Cognitive deficits can be an effect of neuroleptic and anticholinergic medications, but may also occur independent of medication effects.

Limited awareness of emotions

Another basic metacognitive ability often lacking in acute, severe psychosis is a limited mental construct for one's own emotions (alexithymia). Individuals with acute, severe psychosis tend to lack awareness of their emotional experience. In addition, emotions that are displayed often appear dysregulated, either as flat or restricted affect, incongruent affect, or periodic mood lability. Further, as with thinking, emotions experienced during a more regressed, acute psychosis may not be recognized as passing states: rather, emotions may be perceived as indications of who a person is rather than what a person feels. For example, an acutely psychotic individual may experience intense anger as all that defines her within a moment, losing awareness of all other characteristics, feelings, thoughts, and experiences that contribute to her self-definition. As her awareness of herself as a complex individual who has thoughts and feelings reconstitutes, she will be better able to experience anger as one aspect to herself, as something discrete, transient, and separate, but related, to her.

Lack of goal-directed behavior

During an acute psychotic episode, actions not only may lack an apparent purpose, but may also appear extremely disorganized. For example, the individual may wear the same clothes repeatedly, wear layers of clothes or make-up, refuse to bathe, and be poorly groomed. Less frequently, catatonia may be displayed. Avolition, described as a negative symptom that pertains to problems with initiating and persisting in goal-directed activities, can remain a problem after an acute episode. Factors such as ongoing cognitive deficits, low motivation, reduced response to social cues, and anhedonia/depression also can interfere with progress in goal-directed behaviors after the acute phase.

Rationale for the SEL model

The extensive and varied effects of severe forms of psychosis described above underscore the need for multi-faceted services for individuals with these problems. Fortunately, as we advance to a biopsychosocial understanding that recognizes the confluence of factors that may contribute to the development of psychosis, there has been a renewed focus on the role of psychological interventions in treatment. For example, cognitive-behavioral therapy (CBT) for psychosis is recommended as part of national treatment guidelines in some countries (e.g., National Institute of Health and Clinical Excellence, 2009). Other interventions, such as family/systemic intervention models and cognitive rehabilitation, have also demonstrated benefits (Ojeda *et al.*, 2012; Pilling *et al.*, 2002; Seikkula *et al.*, 2011). Interventions to enhance the sense of self, by broadening the self-view and increasing the capacity for metacognition, are also showing promise (Lysaker *et al.*, 2010).

Now, refinement is needed to increase participation and retention, the number of individuals who respond, and the extent to which individuals respond. An important part of refinement is determining the appropriate timing of different interventions. Certainly, rigid adherence to a single treatment approach, without regard to the individual's immediate status, can result in clinical deterioration. This is particularly true with respect to determining when the individual is ready to directly address emotionally difficult issues and express related affect (i.e., do "processing" work). Mental health clinicians often are trained to elicit affect in therapy in order to connect emotions (often of painful experiences that are being avoided or denied) with current difficulties and distress. This is beneficial for the higher functioning client who has the psychological resources to manage affect at the time, but potentially overwhelming or even dangerous for the person not psychologically capable. As an example, one man with acute, severe psychosis, who was being encouraged in therapy to talk about his abusive mother and his feelings about her, informed the therapist, "I hope my voices don't tell me to put my hands around your neck and choke you." The inappropriate timing of the intervention was highly threatening to the person to an extent that increased psychosis and aggressive impulses. It also is not uncommon to prematurely intervene with cognitive interventions that target a person's thoughts before the person has sufficient awareness of existence, let alone of his/her thoughts, and this, too, can result in increased distress and exacerbations in psychosis.

Individuals may benefit more from many of the current treatment interventions once they have better engaged in the therapy and have progressed to a certain level at which arousal is sufficiently reduced, sense of the self is more defined, and there is a capacity to examine thoughts. For example, research has indicated that many cognitive rehabilitation interventions may not only be ineffective when the client is severely inattentive (such as when acutely distressed), but may result in clinical deterioration (Silverstein *et al.*, 2001), highlighting the importance of carefully dosing the intensity and nature of such interventions based on the individual's cognitive status. As another example, it is likely that individuals would be more responsive to social skills training once they are less distressed and self-focused, and, therefore, better able to notice and respond to others. Indeed, there is strong evidence that basic cognitive processing abilities are necessary in order for individuals diagnosed with schizophrenia to learn and respond to psychosocial interventions and to progress in social and vocational functioning (Brekke *et al.*, 2005). Furthermore, individuals with severe psychosis can fluctuate in presentation in terms of reality testing, level of self and interpersonal awareness, cognitive ability, emotional awareness, and arousal level, even within a single meeting. Such variations may affect response to different psychosocial interventions, which underscores the necessity of treatment being flexibly determined by patient status rather than by treatment method. As Fenton (2000) stated, "The crucial question becomes, 'Which interventions are of potential value for a particular individual at a particular phase of illness?'"

To address these issues, a three-phase, conceptual framework was developed that incorporated characteristics of severe psychosis into a dimensional, recovery model in order to select interventions according to client presentation (Fuller, 2009). The SEL model is a practice-based model originally configured from the clinical and empirical literature for psychological interventions for psychosis and refined over time based on the experience of professionals in inpatient and outpatient settings. It was originally implemented in an outpatient psychosocial rehabilitation program of a state psychiatric hospital in the United States, with participation and feedback across diverse professional disciplines, including psychology, nursing, psychiatry, social work, occupational therapy, and recreational therapy. It later was expanded to determine group assignment and types of group interventions for inpatient and outpatient persons served in day treatment of that same setting.

Three phases of psychosis are outlined in the model: Surviving, Existing, and Living. The phases are differentiated by where the individual falls on a continuum of eight different factors: self-definition (i.e., awareness of self as a separate, defined being), interpersonal awareness, threat appraisal, extent of hallucinations or delusions, awareness of thoughts, logical thinking/speech, emotional awareness, and goal-directed behavior. An individual's placement within a phase reflects his or her immediate psychological state, with recognition that individuals may move gradually or rapidly across the continuum, regressing or advancing. This dimensional assessment of multiple, critical factors along a continuum increases precision in determining client status, which then can hone selection of appropriate interventions. Because the SEL model was developed specifically for the most severe forms of psychoses, including schizophrenia, the phases and characteristics within them will be more easily recognized in some individuals with psychosis than others, and not all individuals will experience every phase. Nonetheless, many of the characteristics, treatment interventions, and timing of interventions described are applicable to treatment for other forms of psychosis as well. In summary, the model offers a strategic approach for addressing concerns across a range of domains and symptoms and allows for modification based on fluctuations in client presentation. The objective is to create a better fit between interventions and client readiness in order to increase participation, retention, and treatment efficacy.

Description of the SEL model: surviving, existing, or living

The features of severe psychosis described above are presented as categories in the three-phase model presented in Table 1.1. These factors were chosen based on areas of concern frequently described in the clinical literature and are assessed dimensionally rather than categorically. Each phase of psychosis, Surviving, Existing, or Living, is determined based on where the individual falls on a continuum for the various characteristics, including the extent of self-definition, the level of perceived threat, interpersonal relatedness, emotional awareness, awareness of thoughts, organized and

Table 1.1 Characteristics of the three phases of psychosis

Dimensions	Surviving	Existing	Living
Self-definition	Undifferentiated self (lack of consistent, cohesive, sense of self)	Emerging sense of self	Differentiated self (more stable sense of self)
Interpersonal awareness	Limited awareness of others	Greater awareness of others	General awareness of others/ increased empathy
Threat appraisal	Constant sense of threat	Tendency to perceive events as threatening	More accurate appraisal of threat
Hallucinations/delusions	Prominent hallucinations/delusions	Less prominent hallucinations/ delusions	Limited distress or impairment from hallucinations/delusions
Cognitive awareness	Limited awareness of thoughts	Increased awareness of thoughts	Increased self-reflection and use of thoughts to guide responses
Logical thinking	Disorganized and/or illogical speech	Increased organized and logical speech	Predominantly organized & logical speech
Emotional awareness	Limited awareness or appropriate expression of emotions	Emerging awareness and appropriate expression of emotions	Increased awareness and appropriate expression of emotions
Goal-directed behavior	Limited adaptive and goal-directed behavior	Emerging adaptive and goal-directed behavior	Increased adaptive and goal-directed behavior

logical speech, and the intensity and interference of psychotic responses (such as hallucinations or delusions).

Of note, many of the factors of the SEL model coincide with concepts of metacognitive capacities, or the increasingly complex ability to think about thinking. In general, as described by Koriat and Goldsmith (1996), there is a progression from having knowledge about one's cognitive abilities ("monitoring") to utilization of this knowledge to guide one's actions ("control"). Lysaker and his colleagues (e.g., Lysaker *et al.*, 2011) have expanded and explored application of metacognitive capacities in individuals diagnosed with schizophrenia, including the relationship between metacognitive abilities and the quality of self-experience. Four levels start with knowledge of one's own mental state (especially awareness of personal thoughts and feelings as part of self-reflectivity), followed by awareness of the mental state of others (as in theory of mind concepts), to a positioning of self in relation to others ("decentration") and, finally, to being able to apply one's knowledge of mental phenomena to guide one's actions ("mastery"). While increasing awareness of self, other, personal thoughts, and emotions can be subsumed under current ideas of metacognitive capacities, the SEL model distinguishes them as separate, but related, factors in order to highlight the individual importance of each as targets of assessment and intervention. In a most regressed state, the person loses awareness of all of those aspects of experience, and each is gradually regained as progress is made.

Models of different stages of psychosis, particularly for schizophrenia, have been previously described. Agius *et al.* (2010), for example, have proposed a model for schizophrenia consisting of three stages to be considered when determining treatment: prodrome, first episode, and chronic phase. The SEL model shares the goal of other staging models of tailoring treatment to phase of psychosis, but is based on specific clinical features along a continuum for those exhibiting overt psychosis. Although the SEL model does not include those in a prodromal phase at this time, treatment prior to overt psychosis is critical, and increasing attention is being paid to this essential part of comprehensive care for reducing severity and improving long-term outcome.

The continuum provided for each characteristic in the SEL model reflects that individuals experiencing psychosis, particularly more severe forms, often display vacillations in different areas, such as in intensity of hallucinations or delusions, and in the extent of self, emotional, cognitive, and interpersonal awareness. Diagnostic classifications of schizophrenia have tended to be categorical and, consequently, have not fully accounted for the different experiences of psychosis. Individuals do not fall neatly into categories of "psychotic" or "not psychotic" or "sick" or "well," but experience distortions to varying degrees. For example, auditory hallucinations may be perceived to be more or less intrusive and more or less distressing and the self-structure may be more or less developed at different times. The continuum in the model accounts for these variations with greater specificity than categorical descriptions. The dimensional perspective also reflects growing recognition that the experience of psychosis can range from more severe forms with significant self-disturbance and limited adaptive functioning to the more self-defined, well-functioning individual who hears voices.

The three phases represent different levels of progress or regression across the different domains. Briefly stated, the Surviving Phase is the most regressed, acute phase. During the Surviving Phase, a person questions existence or perceives himself to be under constant threat of harm and may readily misperceive innocuous experiences as threats. As a result, there is a persistent, relentless terror of either not existing or soon perishing. Once personal existence and relative safety are established, the individual moves into an Existing Phase, where there begins some cautious venturing out, psychologically, interpersonally, and physically. As boundaries for the self and between the self and others are better established, there can also be more awareness and interaction with others. Emotional, interpersonal, and intrapersonal experiences may be engaged in very cautiously and in limited ways, which results in a restricted existence. The goal of treatment is to help individuals move into the Living Phase, where it feels safe to engage more fully with the world, to experience a full range of emotions, to try new activities, to introspect in a deeper way, and to participate in closer, more meaningful relationships. The Surviving, Existing, and Living Phases subdivide the range of psychotic experience into three general psychological states, and are considered more loose distinctions than discrete, rigid categories. At any given time, individuals with psychosis may fit best with one phase, but may show characteristics of improvement or decline of other phases.

Overview of interventions

The SEL model provides a framework for determining the phase in which an individual is functioning. Determining the phase then facilitates understanding of particular issues and capacities at that moment which, in turn, can guide the type and timing of interventions to which the person is most likely to be responsive. Examples of goals and types of interventions within each phase are presented in Table 1.2. As an example, in the Surviving Phase, an objective of all interventions is to "fortify" the individual, both in terms of self-experience as well as in bolstering psychological resources for coping in a more direct, adaptive, reality-based manner. This also highlights that the Surviving Phase avoids interventions that may increase psychological distress, such as processing of emotionally provoking topics. Interventions also target increasing a sense of self (differentiation) and of safety in existence. In addition, as part of crucial reality orientation efforts at the most regressed end of the spectrum, interventions in the Surviving Phase emphasize the present more than the past and the future. Group therapies in the Surviving Phase tend to be more activity-based, rather than process-oriented or psycho-educational groups. Normalization of the individual's experience may be received better than teaching, which is easily perceived as efforts to overtake or control the person. The fundamentals of emotion identification and increasing awareness of thoughts lay the foundation for interventions in the Existing and Living Phases. Mental health services in the Surviving Phase are tailored to achieve these objectives, with a particular emphasis on self-definition and safety, including within the therapeutic relationship. Psycho-education for the family is an important part of developing a supportive network for the individual and preparing for possible

Table 1.2 Phase-specific interventions

Surviving	Existing	Living
Fortifying	Continued fortifying/ limited uncovering	More uncovering/ processing
Self-defining work (differentiating)	Self-defining and self-other work	Self-other work (collaborating)
Present focus	Present and future focus	Past, present, and future focus
Activity-based groups	Vocational ("work") therapy	Work
Normalization	Psycho-education/skill building	Psycho-education/skill building
Label and contain emotions	Increase awareness and management of emotions	Encourage more emotional expression
Increase awareness of thoughts	Cognitive-behavioral therapy	Cognitive-behavioral therapy
Psychodynamic therapy (modified)	Psychodynamic therapy	Psychodynamic/other explorative therapies
Collaborative psychopharmacology	Collaborative psychopharmacology	Collaborative psychopharmacology
Psycho-education for families	Psycho-education for families/family therapy	Family therapy

family therapy. Efforts also are made in the Surviving Phase to improve self-care (i.e., activities of daily living) and increase purposeful, goal-directed behaviors.

As the individual moves into the Existing Phase, there is an emerging sense of self, and a growing awareness of emotions, of thoughts, and of others. Interventions continue to fortify the self-structure, heighten awareness of the emotional experience, and improve coping with stressors. More of the person's strengths and aspirations can be elicited in this phase to develop personal goals of recovery. Employment opportunities also may be explored in the Existing Phase. Vocational therapists can assist the client in finding appropriate jobs, help with application and interview preparation, and provide on the job support and supervision. Some limited exploration of emotionally laden topics ("uncovering") may be introduced, with close monitoring of the person's ability to adaptively manage the topic and his/her responses. Both the present and the future are explored, with reference to the past to the extent tolerated. Psycho-education, particularly related to psychosis, stress, and skill building, are important aspects of treatment in the Existing Phase. Additionally, given that cognitive-behavioral interventions for psychosis have been found to be more effective with those who have some awareness of their difficulties (Silverstein *et al.*, 2006), individuals in the Existing Phase may be more responsive to such strategies. A client may be better able to participate in family therapy, particularly sessions that limit emotional expression or exploration of highly emotionally charged issues and focus instead on information exchange, support, coping skills, and improved communication. Psychodynamic therapy in the Existing Phase facilitates understanding of the individual's presentation and experience, intervenes to promote differentiation and strengthening of the self-structure, increase awareness and adaptive expression of emotional experiences, and uses the therapy relationship to effect change. Both psychodynamic and cognitive therapies begin to assist the individual in making meaning of the hallucinations and delusions and in reducing related distress.

In the Living Phase, where there is more awareness of self and others and greater psychological and cognitive capacity to explore emotionally provoking topics, interventions may look more like those for "higher functioning" individuals. For example, the clinical concept of "uncovering" refers to interventions that move from surface to depth, from conscious to deeper issues of the unconscious, and encourage the expression of affect. This is on the far end of the continuum in the Living Phase, when the person has the psychological resources to manage and respond to these kinds of interventions. Generally, such interventions for those with severe forms of psychosis in the Living Phase are conducted cautiously, with attunement to the client's ability to tolerate stress from external and internal challenges. That is, interventions must balance between fortifying and uncovering depending on the individual's immediate status. This is in keeping with efforts to gradually reduce the use of avoidance and denial, which individuals with psychosis frequently employ, and promote the use of more direct, adaptive means of coping (i.e., reduce "sealing over" coping strategies and increase "integration" strategies, McGlashan *et al.*, 1977). Past, present, and future can be navigated with greater tolerance, and the person is more capable of exploring the past as a contributor to the present.

In the Living Phase, both cognitive behavioral and psychodynamic therapies work to increase awareness of the relationship between past and current stressors and psychotic symptoms. Honing of coping skills, increasing self-management of mental health problems, further development of a balanced, satisfying self-identity, and of meaningful relationships are important objectives in this phase. Traumatic experiences proceeding as well as following psychotic experiences also can be further addressed in the Living Phase. Process-oriented group therapies may be beneficial, although skill-building groups remain bedrocks of group interventions for those with severe forms of psychosis in the Existing and Living Phases because of the many skill deficits and interpersonal difficulties. Individuals in the Living Phase may work in the community, but continue to benefit from problem-solving and skill building related to vocational issues. Family therapy may gradually address more difficult and emotionally provoking issues as the individual and the family have the resources to tolerate the challenges. Collaboration between medication prescribers and therapists is critical throughout the phases to allow for coordination of the types of medications needed with the psychosocial interventions being conducted as the individual moves between phases, sometimes advancing and sometimes regressing. Such collaboration can help to maximize responsiveness to psychosocial interventions and psychotherapy.

An important note is necessary with regard to intervention with hallucinations and delusions. Often, treatment professionals assume that reduction of hallucinations and delusions is a goal of intervention that is shared by the client. However, it should not be automatically assumed that the person wishes to eliminate voices or change a delusional belief. One experience-based expert, in commenting on the SEL model, emphasized that a goal to eliminate hearing voices may not be an achievable one and that it also may not be desired. Some delusions and hallucinations are experienced positively, such as when religious explanations are made for the experiences or when voices provide companionship, support, or helpful guidance. Clearly, individuals develop a relationship with their voices over time (Benjamin, 1989) that may be more positive, negative, or neutral in valence. Therefore, initial treatment planning and assessment must include inquiries into the client's level of distress about the voices or beliefs and degree of impairment related to the experiences. Eliciting the client's perspective on what it would be like to be without the hallucinations or to alter a particular unconfirmed belief is also essential in assessment. This fundamental inquiry will reveal crucial information about the individual's perspective and level of insight, level of motivation for change, as well as what the experiences provide for the person. Ultimately, in many contemporary models, goals of recovery target reducing the distress and the interference in functioning experienced due to hallucinations and delusions, rather than elimination of hallucinations and delusions. A person may want to continue hearing positive voices or retain aspects of their beliefs and, particularly if it does not pose safety issues, this circumstance then necessitates that the *mental health professional* change his/her expectations and beliefs instead. This highlights the larger issue that, ultimately, services need to be guided by the individual's goals, with the professional working collaboratively with the client to increase the sense of influence (agency) over his/her life. Having a sense of influence in treatment decisions creates the foundation for building a sense of agency in other aspects of the person's life.

Additionally, Table 1.2 presents some of the important goals and interventions in treating psychosis across the three phases, but it is not exhaustive. Professionals from different disciplines involved in the treatment of psychosis, including nursing, social work, occupational therapy, and recreation therapy, have also used the SEL model to guide their interventions according to the phase in which their client is functioning. While some of the goals listed in Table 1.2 are targeted by many disciplines, there also are service-specific goals not listed that are an important part of recovery. The table may serve for each therapeutic service as a template upon which discipline-specific goals and interventions can be added.

For the model to be implemented within a service agency, it is helpful to have staff across disciplines who are skilled in a range of services and can flexibly provide what the client needs and wants, depending on the phase of psychosis. Whenever possible, having the agency provide care across the continuum minimizes change for the client. Even when the service agency is more focused on individuals within a particular phase (e.g., those with acute, severe psychosis), being able to rapidly identify and intervene when the individual shows signs of regression or progress can minimize adverse change, promote progress, and maintain continuity in care. As an example of agency application of the SEL model, Chapter 6 describes its implementation in outpatient and inpatient units of a psychiatric hospital setting.

With progress and regression, individuals may sometimes fall between two phases, posing a challenge in determining which phase and what interventions would be best to use. In those situations, a best-fit determination is made that attempts to expand a person's abilities without overwhelming current capabilities. In addition, although the person may primarily fit in one designated phase, the astute therapist rapidly adjusts interventions according to where the client is functioning in the immediate moment. That is, after an initial determination of the phase that a person is in, continuous assessment during interventions needs to occur to determine where the individual falls on the continuum for each factor. This is particularly important given the rapid fluctuations that can occur for individuals in brief periods of time. That is, within a single therapy session, an individual may display some of his most regressed functioning as well as portend the higher functioning of which s/he is capable. For example, a client may be describing himself in a reality-based way, then suddenly revert to delusional material where his ideas seem diffuse, confused, and distorted. Such a shift reflects a change in his thinking and of his perception of self and other and signifies a regression from the Existing Phase to the Surviving Phase. The therapist would need to revert to more supportive and fortifying techniques to reinforce and re-establish the individual's sense of existence, separateness, and safety before returning to more exploratory work. In this manner, the SEL model provides a dimensional framework for obtaining more specific information about client status and tailoring interventions accordingly.

Adjustments occur in the nature of the therapeutic relationship concomitant with changes in the individual's presentation, particularly related to trust and intimacy. That is, gradations of interpersonal connection occur across the phases. In the Surviving Phase, where there tends to be an inward focus with little awareness of others, the therapist may often feel as if s/he doesn't exist either, as if invisible to the client. The emphasis at that time is on "differentiating," on being clear about differences between the self and others. As the individual feels more assured about self and safety and spends more time externally focused, s/he may start to let others "in." In the Living Phase, there can develop more of a sense of a therapeutic partnership, of two individuals working together. However, as fluctuations in status occur for the individual, the level of trust and connectedness alters as well, necessitating adjustments in approach by the therapist to maintain an appropriate stance to which the client can respond. Adjustments in the therapeutic relationship according to phase are discussed in subsequent chapters.

The more thorough the case formulation, the more precision there can be in matching treatment interventions to client presentation. Greater understanding of the client also enhances the therapeutic relationship with any service provider. The eight factors described in the SEL model can be used to develop a general conceptualization. The initial formulation then can be expanded through initial information from the client, previous treatment providers, family and other supports, prior records, and other collateral information. Such information provides insight into pre-psychosis functioning and may indicate precipitating factors (including traumatic events) that have contributed to the development of the psychosis. Historical data also assist in determining the highest level of functioning that the individual has achieved, including socially, academically, vocationally, and psychologically. Psychologically, what is the highest level of defenses that the person has utilized? For example, has the person been able to utilize intellectualization, sublimation, and other higher-order defenses? In addition, what does the person's internal template of relationships look like? Transference issues that arise and counter-transference responses that are engendered in each of the three phases provide hypotheses about the client's self–other representations and experiences. Such data from therapeutic encounters, in addition to history, assist in determining predominant personality style. Together, knowledge of the individual's primary psychological defenses, personality structure, and object relations adds necessary depth to the case formulation. The reader is referred to the many excellent resources available that cover these topics in depth (e.g., McWilliams, 1994; Kernberg, 1995).

Many standardized, valid test measures for assessing delusions and hallucinations, personality patterns, and psychological issues exist, although these generally are not valid until the individual with psychosis is sufficiently stabilized. Therefore, although some of the information described above may be available during the first encounter with the client and will provide an initial, working hypothesis, much of the formulation develops over time based on the person's presentation, the issues that arise within and outside of the therapy relationship, and information that emerges from the client and collateral over time and across phases.

Conclusions

Severe forms of psychosis are complex conditions that can disrupt every aspect of an individual's life, down to fundamental facets of the self and of existence. The three-phase, SEL model offers a means for assessing and describing individuals with psychosis along a continuum, from the most regressed aspects of the Surviving Phase to movement into recovery of the Living Phase. Conceptualizing features on a continuum/dimension rather than as discrete categories more precisely represents the fluid nature of psychological status and functioning. Additionally, the greater specificity of the features and issues delineated within each phase can facilitate effective pacing of interventions. As such, the model allows for integration of the many effective therapies in use into a comprehensive approach to care. This approach maintains alignment between therapeutic interventions and client readiness, creating an attunement that facilitates understanding, trust, and effective interventions. From this foundation, a therapist and client can address the problems in living created by severe forms of psychosis in an optimistic, progressive manner that conveys hope for moving away from an "artificial life" to a more genuine and satisfying life experience.

Chapter 2

The Surviving Phase
Characteristics and care

Client:	Can I ask you something?
Therapist:	Of course.
Client:	Am I dead? I think that I went to the dead world.
Therapist:	No, you are alive. I see you in front of me. Can you feel your pulse, your heart beating? That tells you that you are alive.

Conceptualizing and treating the more severe psychoses is a daunting task. First, an acute psychosis for this subgroup displays in full color a terrifying experience of self-dissolution, of losing touch with reality and logic and, ultimately, with existence. The state of high distress and illogical thinking, particularly during an acute episode, makes it difficult – and sometimes unsettling – to comprehend what the person is experiencing. To grasp the experience fully, one has to walk in dark psychological places that we usually make great efforts to avoid.

The intense "ontological insecurity" (Laing, 1960) experienced by the individual in acute-phase, severe psychosis is a distinguishing feature of the disorder and necessitates modification of traditional approaches for successful engagement and treatment. In particular, one of the primary goals of therapy for severe psychosis needs to be enhancement of the sense of a defined, autonomous self who is separate from, but also related to, others (Bachmann *et al.*, 2003). That is, an essential goal is to facilitate differentiation. Accomplishing this goal requires adjustments in the therapist's approach in order to facilitate self-definition and development without heightening core, primitive fears of being overtaken or annihilated. This chapter first describes the unique features of the client and the therapy in the Surviving Phase and then delineates specific interventions for an acute phase of severe psychosis.

Unique characteristics of the person in the Surviving Phase

The unique presentation and concerns of the individual in acute-phase, severe psychosis, both in a first episode as well as chronically, underscores the need to facilitate differentiation. Differentiation in this context refers to the process of increasing an individual's experience of him or herself as a distinct, separate, and cohesive person.

The primary struggle of individuals with severe psychosis is a perceived threat to their existence, what Karon and Vandenbos (1981) referred to with schizophrenia as "existential terror" and Sass and Parnas (2003) identify as an "ipseity disturbance," a diminished awareness of one's existence. This is reflected poignantly in one client's statement, "It's just so damn hard to be." A person needs to know that she exists before she can worry about being killed and psychotic individuals may fluctuate between a fear of annihilation and, when further regressed, a fear that they do not exist. This disintegration of the fundamental self-structure results in, as Andreasen (1999) described, "an inability to distinguish between the self and not-self." The clinical observation that individuals diagnosed with schizophrenia in the most regressed, acute psychotic states seem to make fewer "I" statements reflects these uncertainties about existence and the lack of a defined sense of self. Progress is evident in acute psychosis when the individual increases in awareness of his/her existence, but experiences it as tenuous, as evidenced by expressed fears of being killed, overtaken, or of disintegrating. One woman, for example, described the left side of her body as "corroding" and stated that she saw dust coming off of her body when taking a bath and noted, "I am dust in the wind."

The experience of a limited sense of a differentiated self in severe psychosis is similar to what Stern (2000) called in the infant an "emerging self." The emerging self is defined by immediate, single thoughts, words, or actions, rather than a consistent, cohesive self. Therefore, the individual believes he *is* his thoughts and feelings of the moment rather than that he is a person who *has* thoughts and feelings.

The lack of self-definition also is reflected in the individual's experience of being permeable, a perception that there is not a barrier that keeps the individual in and others out. This can be either a physical and/or a cognitive experience. Physically, it may manifest in such fears as of being transparent, easily invaded, or fused with others (PDM Task Force, 2006). A man who stated that he had "no skin" highlighted the primitive experience of being permeable, with nothing keeping him in and nothing protecting him to keep other things or people out. Others believe that foreign objects have been placed in their body or their brain. Often acutely psychotic individuals experience the body as an external, foreign object rather than as a connected part of the self. For example, one man was encouraged to observe his hands as part of efforts to reassure him that he was alive. He stated, "I can look at my hands, but I don't feel like they are mine." The perception of one's organs falling out also reflects this diffuse state. Such experiences indicate a lack of crucial awareness of the body as a part of the self and as a protective barrier, which are part of the sense of physical cohesion that Stern (2000) described as a requisite aspect of developing a "core self" in the infant.

Similarly, individuals in an acute phase lack awareness of thoughts as a discrete, private aspect of the self. This cognitive permeability is characterized by an absence of awareness or ownership of one's thoughts and a lack of distinction from the thoughts of others. One client described the experience of others reading his mind, including while he was reading, as an experience of continually being "trespassed upon." This can be manifested in uncertainty about whether one actually has thoughts, is his thoughts, possesses other people's thoughts (i.e., thought insertion), or gives away one's thoughts (thought broadcasting). Permeability also is reflected in beliefs that their "bad" thoughts and feelings will affect others and make them bad as well, as if they are contagious. Further, cognitive permeability contributes to the misattributions of thoughts/inner experiences to external sources (i.e., hallucinations), a concept historically considered to occur through the unconscious and anxiety-based mechanism of projection (e.g., Feigenbaum, 1936), with more recent efforts to incorporate this concept into cognitive approaches with the term "faulty source monitoring" (Frith, 1992). Fear of others being able to read one's own thoughts also reflects cognitive permeability. As elucidated by Sass and Parnas (2003), the energy and effort that are focused on what are normally fundamental assumptions outside of conscious awareness (particularly assumptions of existence, of being connected to the body, and of being a person who has thoughts) interfere with spontaneous and automatic cognitive processing, a common deficit for those diagnosed with schizophrenia (Frith, 1979; Gray *et al.*, 1991). A related line of research indicates that individuals diagnosed with schizophrenia often demonstrate compromised metacognitive ability, particularly a limited ability to monitor or self-reflect on one's own cognitive processes (Frith, 1992; Koren *et al.*, 2006) and this correlates with a diminished self-experience (Lysaker *et al.*, 2008).

Interpersonally, the lack of implicit awareness of existence in psychosis results in a hyperfocus inward that prevents awareness of others, a process that Freud (1924/1962) described as a withdrawal of object cathexis. In essence, the basic preconditions for more advanced self-experience and interaction with others, such as innate knowledge of one's existence and of being a prescient, feeling being, are absent or diminished in the individual with acute severe psychosis. Clearer self-definition, including improved physical cohesion and psychological boundaries, must be established first before interacting with another can occur. As the emerging self develops, there can increasingly be an outward focus. However, while a sense of permeability remains, fear persists that closeness with others will result in a loss of identity and of the boundary between the person and the world (Fromm-Reichmann, 1952). Therefore, the process of differentiation generally is marked by periods of more awareness and interaction with others and with surroundings countered by, often sudden, retreats inward.

Unique characteristics of care in the Surviving Phase

The severe self-disturbance of acute-phase severe psychosis, characterized by the lack of implicit awareness of existence, physical and cognitive permeability, and lack of awareness of others, necessitates focusing therapeutic services first on the establishment of a more coherent self in the client before other therapeutic interventions can be effective. This makes sense developmentally, given that awareness of existence precedes awareness of thinking. Consistently, for the individual in an acute psychotic regression, reassurance of existence is a prerequisite for the metacognitive capacity to examine thoughts. Further, a more defined sense of one's self is required to be able to examine thoughts as passing states rather than as an immediate, global characterization of who one is. Interpersonal awareness is also predicated upon having sufficient enough reassurance of existence to be able to focus externally on others. That is, the formation of the senses of a "core self" and "core other" are necessary prerequisites to experiences of "self-being-with-other" (Stern, 2000).

Our increasing understanding of the unique features of acute psychosis has prompted concomitant modifications in clinical approach. Early in the clinical literature, Federn (1934) observed that traditional psychoanalysis tended to exacerbate psychosis for the individual with schizophrenia. He recommended sitting face to face, avoiding "uncovering" of deeper unconscious issues, addressing only what was presented, strengthening the ego, and involving the family in treatment. Since that time, various approaches for promoting self-development have been described, with some emphasizing the need for "therapeutic symbiosis" as a type of corrective experience necessary to form a separate self (e.g., Mahler and Furer, 1960; Searles, 1965) while others have emphasized that the therapy relationship must minimize the risk of intensifying the individual's fears of incorporation (Lidz and Lidz, 1952) and promote independence to avoid remaining in "pathological collusion" (Robbins, 1993). More recently, Lysaker *et al.* (2007) have described fostering a coherent self by facilitating reconstruction of the client's personal narrative, primarily through reflective techniques that emphasize the individual and different aspects and roles of the self.

Each of these approaches reflects different notions about the most effective therapeutic stance, from one of symbiotic fusion with the client to emphasizing greater boundaries between self and other. Refinement in approach, however, necessitates constantly adjusting the therapeutic position based on the client's level of self-development, which often fluctuates considerably during an acute phase. Specifically, in a most regressed state, when the individual is uncertain of his existence, an emphasis on differentiation is important to support the individual in the realization of being a separate, sentient being. Fostering differentiation requires reassurance of existence and safety in existence, increasing awareness of personal characteristics, reconnecting of the self within the body, and reinforcement of the boundary between self and other. As the self-structure develops, greater use may be made of the therapeutic relationship to effect change. The remainder of the chapter describes strategies for accomplishing these tasks in acute-phase psychosis.

Treatment strategies for the Surviving Phase

Engage the client in the therapy

Although this is an obvious objective of treatment, it is often not readily achieved with those experiencing psychosis. Establishing enough rapport to initiate a working, therapeutic relationship is always the first goal of therapy and, with higher functioning individuals in outpatient settings, this is generally more easily accomplished. The individual comes seeking assistance and s/he has enough sense of a separate self, ego strength, and adequate expectation of the therapist as a helper to remain and engage for the therapy hour. For those with more of a borderline organization, much of the therapy may be focused on addressing the therapeutic relationship as it relates to prior experiences and maladaptive relational patterns. The level of rapport may vary dramatically from intensely engaged to significantly detached, but with the relationship – in various forms – remaining.

In working with those with a psychotic organization, however, establishing a relationship that feels safe enough for the person to even enter a therapy room can be significantly challenging. Initially, the person may be so withdrawn into his or her psychotic world that the individual may not even acknowledge a therapist. In addition, as previously mentioned, the lack of differentiation between self and other for the acutely psychotic individual means that even the most benign encounter can be experienced as a terrifying threat of being overtaken or annihilated. For example, one man diagnosed with chronic schizophrenia was generally mute aside from a few occasional words and single sentences. He would, with considerable effort and anxiety, muster up and expel a "hello" when greeted. It was as if he briefly emerged from within his world to engage and then would quickly retreat. Insufficient organizational and adaptive skills during acute psychosis also can interfere with the ability to schedule and present to an office for an appointment.

Given the lack of sense of self, trust issues, and functional impairments, it may take considerable time before a client agrees to meet in an office. Therefore, therapeutic contacts may first involve just greeting the client, gradually moving into more of a conversation, and eventually encouraging the client to attend an office appointment. This means sometimes extending the "frame" of psychotherapy (Langs, 1973) from inside the office to contacts and conversations outside the office, which can occur in day treatment settings, inpatient facilities, community centers, medical offices, and home-based visits. Descriptions of "befriending" the psychotic individual as part of initial engagement (Kingdon *et al.*, 1989), which involves a focus on more neutral topics, a nonconfrontational, accepting approach, and utilization of some self-disclosure to facilitate engagement, reflects growing awareness of the need to modify the traditional approach to engagement when working with those with psychosis. "Befriending," however, is not to be misconstrued as developing a friendship with a client in the way one would with someone outside of a therapeutic relationship, where there would be reciprocal support and disclosure and potential attendance at social activities together. The goal with the individual with psychosis is to create enough safety for the individual to engage, which necessitates a supportive, accepting approach that is less agenda-driven and flexible enough to begin and return to a focus on more benign topics as needed. Self-disclosure is used with caution and only if it may assist in normalizing and engaging. Sessions may initially be five minutes and increase over time as the client is able to tolerate it. This type of engagement is more feasible in residential and day treatment settings, and poses greater challenges in outpatient settings where there is less opportunity for informal contact.

Time spent discussing less emotionally provoking subjects, what may feel like "chatting," is not therapeutically avoidant as might be the case with higher functioning clients. Rather, it is part of helping the client to define herself, fortify boundaries between self and other with less emotionally provoking discussion, give opportunities to increase social interaction and comfort, and allow for reality-based focus. This fits with the emphasis there has been on supportive psychotherapy for individuals diagnosed with schizophrenia in which the goal is "covering" rather than "uncovering." That is, the objective is to fortify defenses (i.e., increase adaptive means of coping) and the sense of self to better manage underlying conflicts, difficult emotions, and memories, rather than reducing defenses to encourage expression of those experiences. This is often a particularly challenging shift for therapists, including new therapists, who are used to working with individuals with greater psychological resources for whom the goal is to increase awareness and expression of emotions, thoughts, and conflicts.

Work with one woman diagnosed with schizophrenia serves as an extreme example of how slow the process of engagement into therapy may be for someone with chronic, severe psychosis and intense mistrust and fear. The woman vacillated for a year between completely ignoring the therapist when greeted and initiating friendly conversations. She stopped into the therapist's office a few times and discussed the office contents, but declined to schedule a time to meet. Eventually, however, she asked if she could sit in the chair just outside the office "when I need to" and later requested to meet with the therapist. After the first time that she sat and talked with the therapist, she subsequently continued to decline set appointments, but requested to see the therapist approximately weekly. It was several more months before she agreed to meet at a regular time. As rapport developed, she started to regularly wait near the therapist's door one to two hours prior to her appointment. Although this example reflects an extreme in the engagement process, it also highlights the need and benefit of persistent, extensive efforts that characterize work with this population.

Create a safe, predictable environment

As with all who have been traumatized and continue to worry that threat of harm remains, it is essential to establish a sense of safety for the individual with severe psychosis. This means actions and words and an environment that indicate that their psychological and physical self will not be harmed during the session. This is particularly important given that rates of traumatic events and posttraumatic stress disorder (PTSD) in schizophrenia have been shown to be equal to or higher than for other mental health disorders. Therefore, for individuals who were previously traumatized by others, enhancing a sense of safety may include distinguishing past threats from current circumstances, emphasizing that the traumatic event is over, and identifying ways that the person is safe in the present. Specific trauma-relevant techniques are described in detail in Chapter 6.

Sometimes it is necessary and helpful to make explicit statements regarding safety, such as stating that the office or other meeting place is safe, that no one will get hurt in that space, and that others cannot hear the conversation. Clarifying the limits of confidentiality (what will be said in written and verbal form and to whom) also is important. If not meeting in an office, allowing the client to choose the meeting area and, thereafter, maintaining that location as a consistent meeting place contributes to safety and predictability. One client requested that the therapist answer the phone if it rang during a session instead of allowing it to go to voicemail or turning the phone off, because he wanted to be assured that the caller could not hear the therapy conversation. Answering the phone felt safer to him than worrying that the caller would intrude and listen in on the session. Clearly and promptly addressing expectations that the therapeutic relationship will recapitulate prior experiences of harm also is essential. For example, a 61-year-old woman with a sexual abuse history seductively rubbed her stomach and asked the female therapist if she wanted to have her (the client's) baby. The therapist responded by clarifying the boundaries of the therapy relationship and reassured her that caring would be conveyed only by talking in the therapy. When paranoid clients escalate in their fear of being harmed and, as a result, start to become threatening, many will de-escalate merely with the acknowledgment that it is clear that they are capable of protecting themselves. This diminishes the perceived threat and bolsters the belief in their ability to maintain their safety. Some clients also appreciate delineating specifically what space is theirs and what is the therapist's to emphasize a physical boundary.

Increase the perception of self as a separate, defined individual

In the initial work with a neurotically organized client, one makes efforts to identify and "join" with the client. However, for a client with severe psychosis, who fears being annihilated or engulfed and has little sense of herself as existing and separate from others, it is important that the initial work focus on enhancing the sense of a defined self as separate and different from the therapist. Before differentiation, the experience is one of diffusion and transparency, such that someone knowing one thing about the client feels as if the therapist knows everything. In addition, until one is better defined, one thought or feeling or action immediately defines the self rather than serves as a brief experience or one aspect of the self. Therefore, it is essential to bolster the sense of self as existing and defined *and* reinforce the self as separate from you *before* exploring thoughts and feelings. In a most regressed psychosis, when energy is focused inward, there is limited awareness of the therapist and so there is limited focus on the therapy relationship. A therapeutic relationship still exists, but emphasizes strengthening boundaries between the client and what is outside of him, including the therapist, rather than reducing barriers. As the individual begins to develop self-cohesion and awareness of existence, awareness of "other" also increases. However, because existence remains tenuous, an "other" can readily be perceived as a threat of merger or annihilation (Laing, 1960; Klein, 1946). As an analogy, for an emerging self, the fear of engulfment by others is akin to being sand on a beach, such that, when waves come up the shore, the sand is overtaken, scattered, and washed away. In contrast, for someone with a better defined sense of self, the experience of encountering others is like that of a well-defined rock. The rock, while it may be somewhat altered over time by waves, maintains its basic form and essence. This fragility in self-definition in the client warrants close attention and modification by the therapist in order to fortify the individual and reduce fears of being "overtaken and scattered."

Highlighting differences between the emerging self and others is an important aspect of allaying such fears and fostering differentiation. For example, one client with chronic severe psychosis started to become more anxious and psychotic when the therapist asked how she was doing. Specifically, she began talking more rapidly, saying such things as, "I am not a psychologist. I don't do that psycho-ology thing." The therapist took a step away from her and said, "You are right. I am a psychologist and you are not. We are two different people." The client then slowed her speech and talked about how the therapist was "getting tan" and she wasn't. The therapist agreed with her and commented how well she (the client) was protecting her body and taking care of herself by covering up when in the sun. In this case, simply asking how the client was doing had felt too encroaching for her. With the separateness of therapist and client reinforced, she was then able to proceed in conversation with demonstrably lower anxiety and without further retreat into psychosis.

In addition to fortifying the boundary between the client and the therapist, clarifying that the mental health professional is separate from others also is an important task. It is quite common for individuals with a distorted perception of threat and porous boundaries to merge the therapist with all others, particularly others whom the individual sees as potentially harmful. It is one of the mental health professional's tasks, therefore, to distinguish him or herself as separate and different from other individuals in the client's past or present. With the neurotic client, this type of transference often is encouraged to develop so that it can be explored and addressed within the therapy. However, the tenuous, vulnerable, and precarious nature of the individual with severe psychosis necessitates prompt, clear, and direct interventions that distinguish the mental health professional from others. For example, statements by the client such as "you guys ..." occur when the client's distrust becomes pervasive enough to include the therapist in the group of dangerous others. At such times, the therapist makes efforts to distinguish him or herself as a separate individual, to return the focus to the immediate therapy relationship, and explore whether there are specific things that the therapist has done to raise concerns by the client. This direct clarification and challenge to the client's paranoid projection within the therapy relationship reduces ambiguity in treatment and reiterates safety, both important goals of treatment for those prone to misperception.

Experiences running a group focused on bolstering self-definition in chronically acute individuals further illustrates the struggles of differentiation and problems with merger. When a client was asked what he thought should be the name for a new group that focused on how each individual is his/her own person, he immediately suggested "who be me but you?" and began to talk in a faster, less logical way. When it was reiterated that the group topic would be about how each person is his own separate individual, different from others, he said, "Like how I'm good at bowling and you are not?" and became calmer and more logical when this was confirmed. On the first day of the group, when asked what rules the group thought would be important, one member immediately looked around and said, "Barriers. We need barriers." These examples reflect the frightening threat of fusion with others and the need to increase the "barriers" that separate individuals in order to contain and protect each person.

Fortifying the experience of a physical self separate from others can include raising an individual's awareness of his or her own body, such as what it looks like and how it provides a protective barrier between what is inside and what is outside. This can be helpful in reducing the feeling of permeability and in enhancing safety and self-definition. Pointing out the client's physical features – similar to the comments made about an infant and toddler (e.g., "What bright, blue eyes she has," admiring an infant's hands, and commenting on a toddler's size), but in a non-infantilizing manner – also facilitates the development and awareness of the self. Additionally, increasing sensory awareness further connects the individual to the body and distinguishes the self from the environment. For example, mindfulness techniques that utilize the five senses to facilitate awareness in the immediate moment assist the client in orienting to the present in a calm and reassuring way. Eliciting and sincerely valuing the individual's preferences, opinions, and ideas also promote self-definition. Another way to increase differentiation is by phrases such as "Oh, I guess we see that differently, which is okay because it just highlights that we are different in some ways and that makes this interesting."

In cases of somatic distortions, education and interventions help the client to perceive physical signs as information that the body needs attention rather than an intrusion from outside the self. For example, an inpatient female attributed her menses to her mother chewing on her uterus, causing her to bleed. A man with prostate problems thought unseen others were causing him pain upon urination. For these individuals, as well as for the man who stated that he had "no skin," it was essential in the therapy to discuss the protective features of the body and assist the individual in understanding typical bodily functions and, when necessary, possible medical symptoms. Such interventions contribute to the foundation necessary for reconstituting a sense of a separate, contained, and protected self.

Begin family work

For first-episode psychosis, intensive efforts to work with the individual and family in the community are demonstrating success (Aaltonen *et al.*, 2011). In some countries, including in the UK, offering family interventions is considered part of standard of care for psychosis (National Institute of Health and Clinical Excellence, 2009). However, concerns related to boundaries/merger and problems in affect regulation can be particularly evident in family interactions, highlighting the need to assess client readiness for family therapy sessions. If the individual is not ready for family sessions, initial family work may involve individual therapy for the client and discussions with family members without the client present. As part of fortifying and instilling trust, the client always needs to be informed of these contacts with family members, with information about what will be discussed and what will remain private. Objectives with the family include collaboration, psycho-education about the nature of the individual's difficulties, identification of stressors for and strengths of the family, and agreement and investment in the client's goals. The more influential the family members currently are in the person's life, the more important it is to have them participate in recovery. The exception is if the family members have been abusive and/or remain so, then the therapeutic intervention becomes one of helping to protect the client.

In addition, brief, structured family participation may help to directly address some of what hallucinations and delusions attempt to resolve or avoid. For example, one woman often spoke of her daughter as if she were still the child she was when the woman was first hospitalized over twenty years previously. She had primarily been hospitalized since that time and had not seen her child during those two decades. She would knit baby and young child clothing items for her daughter and request to send them. Maintaining the belief that her daughter was still a child and knitting for her defended against the grief and loss she experienced in not being in her daughter's life. With the help of the case manager, the therapist was able to contact the adult daughter and make plans for renewed contact. The daughter previously had declined contact but now – with information about her mother as well as her current life circumstances – felt more ready to reinitiate contact. Individual sessions focused on preparing the client for talking with her daughter. She was anxious about making contact and tended to express it somatically, such as "I can't hear well, so I don't know what to say" and frequently reported not feeling well. The therapist and client wrote out specific topics that could be discussed and developed a sign that the client could use to inform the therapist if she needed a break during the phone call. The therapist was present during the call to help facilitate as needed and to provide support. Use of the telephone provided an additional barrier to increase the woman's initial comfort level with the interaction. The client, who frequently spoke to unseen others and often was delusional in conversation, was oriented and logical when talking with her daughter. She displayed tears of joy after talking with her daughter and learning that she was going to be a grandmother. With recommencement of the relationship in the present, there was no longer a need to maintain a delusion of her daughter as a child in order to be connected to her. Current excitement about being a grandmother also helped to ease some of the grief and loss of time with her daughter in the past.

In summary, family work in the Surviving Phase concentrates on identifying family stressors that contribute to current difficulties and facilitating involvement of and collaboration with relevant family members, while strengthening the individual as a distinct and separate individual. To achieve these ends, this may mean separate interactions with family members from sessions with the client or brief, structured meetings with family members present.

Promote awareness of thought processes

The initial cognitive work during the Surviving Phase involves facilitating the individual's fundamental awareness of thoughts as a distinct aspect of the self-experience. The individual's abilities to distinguish thoughts from the self and to think about thinking are essential prerequisites for responding to subsequent interventions targeting thoughts and perceptions and their relation to feelings, actions, and hallucinations and delusions. The ability to distinguish thoughts and feelings from the self has mediated response to cognitive interventions with depression (Teasdale *et al.*, 2002) and may improve treatment response for those diagnosed with schizophrenia (Silverstein *et al.*, 2006).

The strategies discussed earlier to enhance a person's self-perception as separate and contained may assist in this development. Educating clients about the transient nature of thoughts and about the frequency of disturbing thoughts in the general population also can assist in normalizing thinking (Kingdon and Turkington, 2005). However, in addition to a diminished or lack of ability to think about thinking, actively psychotic individuals often avoid introspection because it brings more attention to auditory hallucinations and to thoughts and beliefs and the related feelings of distress. Therefore, discerning thoughts from voices heard, and emphasizing how awareness of personal thoughts can help to decrease any stress experienced, can enhance willingness to examine thoughts. Beginning to assess specific details about the hallucinations or delusional beliefs in itself provides the individual with an experience of attention and exposure to distressing voices and ideas, thereby reducing avoidance and diminishing the power and threat of the experiences.

In addition, when clients report what their voices say, the therapist can respond with, "but what does your own voice say?" This is an important step in acknowledging thoughts as well as beginning to explore and assess when the client has commensurate beliefs/thoughts/feelings as the projected "voice," and whether she wishes to agree with or respond to the external information. Questioning how life would be without the distressing voices or particular beliefs introduces a challenge to the certainty and permanence of the hallucinations or delusions. It also provides information about the meaning and purpose these experiences provide. Counting the number of thoughts and gentle, in-session tests of cognitive permeability also may prove useful. For example, one client expressed a fear that the therapist could control his mind. The therapist, having frequently and unsuccessfully encouraged the client to attend groups, said, "Well, if I could control your mind, you'd be going to groups."

Delusional beliefs present a particularly difficult challenge for assessment and intervention. The first challenge is to determine whether a belief truly qualifies as a delusion in need of intervention. The broad, general definition of a delusion is as a false belief. A variety of qualifiers have been added to the definition in efforts to distinguish it from non-pathological beliefs, such as a belief that is inconsistent with ordinary life experience, a belief that lacks confirming evidence, and/or a belief that is inconsistent with cultural norms. However, even with such qualifiers, these definitions continue to include ideas that are not considered pathological. For example, many people believe in such things as UFOs and aliens, which are outside of ordinary life experience, lack supportive evidence, and are not consistent with cultural norms. Religious beliefs also can pose a challenge as religious ideas may or may not be considered delusional. For example, some individuals believe that God has chosen them to do certain things and/or to be special in some way. Societal response and cultural beliefs clearly influence whether such experiences are perceived to be pathological or divine. If enough people believe that person, then it is likely to elevate him or her to a person of religious stature rather than result in admission to a hospital.

Ultimately, it is not so much the nature of the belief that determines pathology as it is the extent to which it interferes with the individual's functioning, including the abilities to carry out activities of daily living, focus on and engage in life, and participate in relationships. Therefore, an essential part of the definition of a delusion is that the belief is held despite a lack of supportive evidence *and* it results in distress for the individual or significantly interferes with the person's functioning. With this approach, beliefs are assessed in terms of the extent to which the individual believes it, the amount of time spent related to the belief, and the extent of negative impact on daily living, with the most severe impairment being deemed delusional and in need of intervention.

Another problem in discerning what is factual from what is part of a delusion or thought disorder is that caregivers and treatment professionals can all too easily dismiss as unfounded and illogical everything an individual with psychosis says that doesn't readily make sense or have confirming evidence. For example, a woman was admitted to a psychiatric hospital due to intense paranoia and regression to a point of living in squalor and being unable to care for herself. Some of her report was unable to be verified (for example, that people were spying on her in her apartment), but this resulted in doubting the veracity of any of her statements. In particular, she was considered to be displaying grandiose delusions when she stated that she was an established author and expert in her field of work, and it was with surprise that her list of professional publications was found on the Internet. Discounting of the individual's ideas, experiences, and sentiments can occur in large and small ways. One outspoken, long-term patient at a state hospital would walk rapidly up and down the hallways cursing the government-employed staff as "(expletive) helots." This usually was a phrase inserted within pressured and extensive rants that were perceived by staff to be illogical ramblings. The term "helots" was dismissed as a neologism. It was with surprise that a psychologist later came across the definition of the word "helot" as an ancient Greek term meaning "state-owned slaves."

Finally, even when none of the content of the psychotic person's speech can be verified, themes and emotions can be conveyed in the meta-communications. As one man said, "When I get sick and talk faster, I may not make sense to you, but I make sense to me." Such examples highlight the importance of mental health professionals avoiding a dichotomous approach that either the client speaks the truth or she doesn't, and be willing to explore the extent to which aspects of the person's speech and beliefs reflect their actual experience or related feelings, thoughts, and concerns.

Thorough exploration of the specific details of the belief initiates the process of determining to what extent and how the belief affects the individual and, therefore, whether it constitutes a delusion that might benefit from collaborative intervention. Eliciting details of the belief can be initiated during the Surviving Phase and continue as the individual progresses. The individual may be reluctant to provide details for many reasons, including expectations that the person inquiring will not believe them. It is, understandably, quite distressing for someone to believe something with certainty, yet have others as adamantly not believe it. Even more difficult is to have others make extensive efforts to convince the person that s/he is wrong and to discount the firmly held belief as a symptom and part of the person's illness. As a result, most clients will assume that the therapist will not believe them and will try to "change their mind." As one client expressed after telling the therapist that he was a four-star general, "You think I am exasturbating." The neologism "exasturbating" appeared to be an amalgam of the words "exaggerating" and "masturbating," which indicated – in part – his awareness that the therapist did not believe his statements. It also reflected his unsuccessful efforts to boost his self-esteem and receive admiration, acceptance, and connection through grandiose statements about himself. His "exaggerating" was only self-stimulating, and left him distanced from others. With that individual and many clients, it takes time to demonstrate that the therapist's intention is to understand the client's perspective and assist in decreasing distress and improving his/her life experience. It is not uncommon for a client to ask the therapist if she or he believes what the client professes. In responding, it is important for the therapist to be honest about his/her perspective and intentions as well as to introduce the notion that there isn't certainty in the idea. For example: "I can see that you believe this, but I am not convinced. We may be seeing it differently, which is fine. It is very important what you believe and how you came to believe it."

Therapists often share the client's reluctance to discuss the details of a problematic belief, but for different reasons. For the therapist, often there is a concern that exploring the belief may convey agreement and collusion with the client, with exploration feeling like reinforcement of the ideas. To avoid this, inquiry requires asking questions in such a way that doesn't suggest agreement, but indicates a desire to understand the individual's perspective. For example, "When did you first start to have the sense that someone was altering your thoughts by manipulating sound waves?" or "I do not know what that experience would be like. Can you describe what that feels like to you?" The difficulty in asking questions in a way that does not suggest full agreement underscores the need to be forthright initially that the therapist may not see the ideas in the same way, but wants to understand the client's perspective.

Another reason for reluctance to explore beliefs on the part of the mental health professional is that therapists and other caring individuals in a delusional client's life can feel compelled to try to convince a client that their belief is false. Although, as previously emphasized, such an approach tends to press the individual into defending beliefs, it can be more uncomfortable and distressing for caring others than for the client to hear the delusional ideas. Certainly, from a pragmatic standpoint, it can seem that, if the person just stopped believing what they do, then there wouldn't be a problem. Some cognitive flexibility on the part of the clinician is required to explore, understand, and address the underlying origins and purposes of the belief. This flexibility requires a shift for most treatment professionals from altering the individual's beliefs to more thoroughly and effectively addressing the reasons for the emergence of the problematic belief for sustained improvement in quality of life and functioning.

In addition to distinguishing thoughts from actions and starting to assess the specific nature of hallucinations and delusions, fundamental cognitive work in the Surviving Phase involves providing clear and, often, frequent reassurance that thoughts are different from actions. One male client was experiencing an increase in paranoia, believing that the police were monitoring his thoughts and that he was going to get into trouble (although he wouldn't say why). Upon exploration of any recent changes or concerns in his life, he mentioned that there was a new female staff member working at the group home where he lived. When asked, "Is she cute?" he looked embarrassed and said that he does not think about such things. When he was informed that he was likely one of the few, and that people often notice if someone is attractive or not and may even have sexual thoughts about them, that this was normal, and that thoughts are private and are different from actions, he subsequently talked more about her and did not report any further concerns about the police monitoring his thoughts. This intervention highlights the importance of normalizing experiences as well as differentiating thoughts and feelings from behavior. In addition to reminding them of the difference between internal experience and action, it can be helpful to reiterate at times that "Your thoughts and feelings are your own, they are private, and others – including me – can only know what you choose to tell." This emphasizes an important boundary between their thoughts and behavior as well as reinforcing the boundary between them and others.

Be clear

When working with neurotically functioning clients, a less directive, generally non-disclosing, and more ambiguous therapeutic stance can be important for addressing issues as they arise within the therapeutic relationship. Questions are often returned to the client to explore his ideas, wishes, and beliefs. In addition, increasing some anxiety in that process may also facilitate change. With the psychotically organized client, however, such ambiguity can actually make the client more psychotic by amplifying distortions and anxiety. Psychotic reactions can be automatic, extreme stress responses to perceived threats and it is the therapist's task to help lessen the sense of threat (in part by increasing the accuracy in appraising threat) and then to assist in developing more adaptive, reality-based means for responding. For example, a client expressed fear that someone was going to hurt her right after hearing loud sounds from outside the therapy office. Simply showing the client the source of the noise and reassuring her of her safety provided the experience of checking facts and more accurately appraising the source of perceived threat. In addition, silence can be too ambiguous and uncomfortable for someone who is actively psychotic, and often it is helpful to specify the reason for being quiet. "I am being quiet right now because I am thinking about what you just said. It is important and I am trying to understand." Specifying movements can also be helpful: "I am going to get up and get something off my desk to show you." These types of interventions are beneficial for reducing fear and distortions for any hyper-vigilant client. In addition, part of "being clear" with paranoid clients is informing them that you cannot read their mind, so you will only know what they are thinking when they choose to tell you. Overall, clarifying intentions, movements, and thoughts help create a clearer, more predictable experience for the client and serve to reduce the sense of threat and increase accurate perception and appraisal.

Limit use of interpretation

Laing (1960) emphasized not expressing too much understanding of a client with schizophrenia, as this can feel intruding or engulfing. Therefore, clarifying rather than interpreting, and bolstering coping rather than challenging defenses, particularly during the early phases of treatment, is advised. Interpretations, particularly genetic interpretations (i.e., interpretations that connect current behaviors or experiences with early experiences), should be paced based on the person's ability to tolerate the information, the accompanying emotions and insight, and the interpersonal closeness that comes with increased understanding. Some interpreting related to current issues may be useful for identifying and clarifying the meaning of what the person is saying, but must be used with caution.

Therapist:	What brought you here to the hospital?
Client:	(*Agitated*) Grief. My children are dead. There was a bomb in [her hometown] and there were bodies everywhere.
Therapist:	Your children feel dead to you. It has been so long since you have seen them.
Client:	Yes. (*Calms down*)

This interpretation merely attempted to clarify by reflecting the emotion of grief that the client was expressing at the loss of contact with her children. Such interpretations, when used judiciously, can increase the individual's awareness of her experience and serve to validate those experiences. However, clarifying through questions rather than statements often is better received, as it allows the individual the opportunity to choose and define his experience rather than having it told to him. Clarifying through questions, then, can enhance self-definition and reduce the experience of feeling intruded upon or engulfed.

Normalize

There are many opportunities in work with individuals with severe psychosis for normalizing their experience, thoughts, and feelings, and discussing adaptive means of expression. Particularly during the initial phase of treatment, however, highlighting how one is similar to others can be very threatening to the person with diffuse boundaries. For similar reasons, therapist self-disclosure as part of normalizing may heighten anxiety for the client because it highlights sameness and takes steps toward closeness with the client that may be perceived as a threat toward merger. In addition, educative efforts by the therapist can be experienced as efforts to impose upon the individual. Therefore, it is important to plan and to be judicious in normalizing and educating in the Surviving Phase, and phrase information in such a way that the individual can choose to relate to it or be different from it. This can further facilitate development of an autonomous identity. For example, saying "I don't know if this is true for you, but many people feel frustrated when someone interrupts them repeatedly" allows the individual to hear that frustration is a normal response to such a situation, but one can choose whether she or he is the same or different.

It is especially important to normalize sexual and aggressive feelings. For example, psychotic clients tend to perceive any aggressive feelings, no matter how mitigated, as potentially being expressed as uncontrolled rage that could result in annihilation of themselves or others. In consequence, feelings of anger may be denied and even mild expressions of discontent avoided. For example, one client noted how hot it had been in a hospital van during a long ride but looked surprised and unsettled when asked why he did not request that staff turn on the air conditioner. He indicated that he would not want to impose on someone else and became visibly anxious when the issue of assertiveness as opposed to aggression was introduced. Even minor assertiveness was perceived as potentially opening the floodgates of rage and, therefore, had to be stifled. However, the denied angry affect and aggressive impulses may be misattributed to others ("people want to hurt me," "you are mad at me") or manifested in hallucinations.

Sexual thoughts and feelings also are frequently of concern. Distress about sexual thoughts and feelings toward the opposite sex as well as the same sex can be intensified for the person with severe psychosis by many issues, including: the tendency to merge sexual feelings with aggression, the belief that anything sexual is bad, fears of fusion with another person, the lack of distinction between thoughts and actions, and fears that others will know their sexual thoughts and feelings. Negative sexual experiences in the past as well as sexual traumas may also contribute to fears. There has been longstanding discussion in the clinical literature that concerns about attraction and intimacy, particularly pertaining to the same gender, can contribute to distress and paranoia (Freud, 1911/1957). Recognition of these areas of concern has been clarified and advanced over the years. For example, Karon and Vandenbos (1981), noting that, developmentally, it is easier to relate first to the same sex, elucidated that what frequently underlies these worries is a longing for closeness that is misperceived as sexual desire. For psychotic individuals with diffuse boundaries, relating to the same or opposite gender can rapidly be equated with merging in a sexual way. Therefore, as themes regarding sexuality become evident, normalizing sexual thoughts and feelings, reassuring that others will only know if the client expresses them, and exploring sexual beliefs and perceptions can help to lessen the associated anxiety. That is, same- and opposite-gender feelings are normalized, with assistance in distinguishing between desire for closeness and sexual desires, as well as recognizing and supporting the client in his/her sexual identity and orientation.

The therapeutic relationship affords many in vivo opportunities for reassurance that aggressive and sexual impulses of the emerging self can be safely addressed, managed, and contained. Intimacy, by nature, can increase both sexual and aggressive feelings, and this is particularly a challenge for those prone to distortion and unable to manage even benign interpersonal and affective experiences. Both erotic and aggressive feelings in general as well as specifically toward the therapist may emerge, necessitating emphasis on the therapist being able to contain such feelings and ensure that impulses, while discussed and normalized, are not acted upon. A woman started out a session in a very pleasant mood, greeting the therapist by saying, "I'm not having any killing feelings in here today." In another example, when a therapist proposed that a client's behavior (saying he hates therapists, saying he felt like hurting someone, saying he can't talk with the therapist about his history) suggested he was upset with the therapist, he said, "I'm not mad at you and I don't want to kill you." Clients may also fantasize and/or worry that the therapy relationship will become a sexual or romantic one. The lack of psychological resources for dealing with these natural impulses highlights the importance of assessing and addressing them in the therapy as the sense of self and the therapeutic relationship develop. Such interventions not only reaffirm safety for both the client and therapist from the client's impulses, but also begin the essential initial work of integration of these expected, but often unwanted, aspects of the self.

Provide increased structure and "containment" when necessary

Notably, when more severely regressed, individuals may need physical containment to prevent acting upon escalating aggressive or sexual impulses. One man stated that, when acutely psychotic, he needed to be somewhere "where I can't control anyone." On occasion, some psychotic individuals struggling with uncontrollable impulses will commit crimes that result in the physical confinement of jail. For example, when reflecting upon his sexual assault crime that occurred during a psychotic episode, a man described that he had escalated to a point of feeling out of control, intentionally committed a crime, and then turned himself in to the police. He noted that he had subsequently experienced relief at being placed in locked confinement "to keep me from myself" and from further acting on his impulses. Ideally, efforts are made to provide this containment in the least restrictive environment for a minimal period of time, with return to the community as soon as clinically indicated. The therapist often serves as the container that Bion (1962) described and this may suffice, at times, for the individual with severe psychosis. Voluntarily wrapping in a blanket or staying alone in a room with minimal stimulation may provide some needed "holding" as well. However, there are times when the physical containment of a day hospital, crisis unit, or inpatient hospital may, temporarily, be necessary. Acute day hospitals, where available, serve this purpose well. Inpatient hospitalization should be used only when other interventions prove insufficient. The goal is always to advance the person to less restrictive settings within her community.

Introduce emotion identification

Psychotherapy typically includes heightening a client's awareness of his/her emotional experience. However, emotion focus with individuals with acute phase severe psychosis often requires more rudimentary and cautious intervention, given the tendency to deny and project unwanted affect. For example, when becoming tearful while discussing missing his recently deceased mother, a client said, "I am not depressed and I have not cried about this. But I am aware that my eyes appear to be relieving themselves." Interventions might start with the primary focus on thoughts before gradually and carefully working on acknowledging emotions, often in a mitigated form that is normalized. For example, "I wonder if you are a little bothered by what John said to you this morning. It certainly would be understandable if you were." Rudimentary awareness of the emotional experience also often requires separating somatic experiences from emotional ones. Stress is often first noticed in the body and somatic concerns provide rich material for exploring what the body might be letting the person know about how he or she is feeling emotionally. For example, one man became increasingly anxious while participating in psychological testing. At one point, he clutched at his chest and said, "My heart! You're killing me, lady." The evaluator said, "People often get kind of stressed during testing and I think feeling your heart beating is letting you know that you are a little stressed. You're okay. Let's just take a break for a minute." Another client's description of having "an emotional cold" when she was feeling sad highlights the merging of somatic and emotional issues that can occur in the more regressed individual. Obviously one needs to assess for signs of true physical concerns before moving to a psychological interpretation, particularly given the myriad of medical problems individuals with severe psychosis can experience.

Continuously monitor and adjust the psychological space in the therapy relationship as needed

As safety in existence develops and awareness of others increases, fears of being overtaken are further complicated by desires for longing and attachment. That is, as the perception of being a separate person becomes implicit, focus and energy can begin to turn outward. It is at these times that the client seems to suddenly become aware of the therapist and ambivalence in the therapy relationship becomes more evident. The individual's struggle with longing for intimacy but fears of merger may be reflected in fluctuations between a rather encroaching engagement with and a schizoid withdrawal from others, what Peciccia and Benedetti (1996) described as vacillations between the symbiotic and separate selves in the person diagnosed with schizophrenia. Such vacillations require that the therapist constantly adjust the therapeutic approach based on the client's status in order to maintain the necessary psychological space between self and other that allows for safe engagement. For example, the client who had felt encroached upon when asked how she was doing, at other times identified ways that she and the therapist were similar. At the onset of the first time she sat down in the office, she made many comments about the office contents, noting that she had some similar items, but of a different color. When she commented on the therapist's shoes looking new, the therapist noted, "Yes, but your shoes [which were the same color as that of the therapist] are much shinier." The client smiled and said, "This is what I want to tell you …" and proceeded to engage in the session. Highlighting differences within the similarities adjusted the psychological distance between her and the therapist, thereby providing safety from merger for her.

Utilize nuances of language

The subtleties of language also can be used to support the client's level of self-development, such as when the therapist adjusts wording based on the level of self-definition and security presented. For example, when the client is most regressed, the therapy is focused primarily on the client and on fortifying a sense of self. Therefore, the therapist may predominantly use the term "you" and encourage the client to make more "I" statements, with very little discussion of the therapist or therapeutic relationship. As a sense of self develops, there may be more of "you" and "I" in comparison, with emphasis on differences between the client and others, including the therapist. Eventually, there is more use of the phrase "You and I," which reassures that there are two, distinct individuals and highlights collaboration without merger. Because "we" is a merger term denoting two people combining into one, use of the term "we" to refer to the client and therapist should be saved for when the client has progressed to a point of being able to join in the therapeutic relationship without feeling the threat of being engulfed. Given the frequent fluctuations in the individual's sense of self, particularly in more regressed psychotic states, the language used to describe the therapeutic relationship often changes within the therapy session as well as across sessions. Similar to the toddler whose confusion of pronoun usage reflects emerging, but confusing, distinctions between self and others, it remains difficult in this period of self-development to be clear where the self ends and the other begins. One client's comments at the end of three different sessions are illustrative of this confusion between self and other. At the end of an early session she said, "Thank you for talking to you." The next week she left saying, "Thank you for talking to myself." A few weeks later she said, "Thank you for talking to me."

Conclusions

Engaging a client with severe psychosis in psychotherapy and other mental health services during an acute phase can be especially challenging and warrants a unique approach that attends to the particular fears and features of the individual at that time. In addition to the longstanding emphasis on supportive therapy, efforts to enhance self-definition and safety are important aspects of psychological treatment for the acutely psychotic individual that warrants further investigation. The emphasis on differentiation in therapy facilitates intimacy without merger, creating the necessary psychological space between self and other that allows for safe engagement. Once the individual is more assured of his existence and safety and begins to display a more consistent, coherent self, the therapist gradually can incorporate more typical ways of connecting with the client. Interventions for that next phase, the Existing Phase, are described in Chapter 3.

Chapter 3

The Existing Phase
Characteristics and care

"I have been paralyzed for a long time and am starting to get some feeling back."

Unique characteristics of the person in the Existing Phase

The Existing Phase is characterized by an increasing awareness of the self and others, which includes an increasing awareness of thoughts, emotions, and of the body, of others, and of the surrounding environment. The individual displays a more consistent sense of self and a more moderate level of arousal. Evidence of this movement into the Existing Phase may include increasing recognition of different aspects to a complex self, displaying an increasing awareness of and interaction with others, and displaying increased tolerance for experiencing stress without immediately regressing into psychotic perceptions and responses. Most individuals continue to experience distressing auditory hallucinations and/or delusions in this phase, but they may be less intrusive and disruptive as they become one part of the person's experience rather than the sole experience. In addition to an overall emerging connection with the self and the world, the concurrent restrictions on experience in the Existing Phase are evident in the efforts to keep aspects of the individual's life simplified in order to function. This is evident in the tendency to minimize the range of experience within the self (emotionally, cognitively, and in self-concept) as well as interpersonally. Great efforts may be made to maintain routine and limit activities. While this may be partially attributable to residual negative symptoms and/or medication side-effects, an additional aspect is the perceived necessity of keeping things simple to avoid becoming overwhelmed.

The mental health clinician likely will discover that there can be a considerable range of functioning within the Existing Phase. Some individuals will seem more tenuous in their sense of self and still require more supportive therapies and fundamental work in consolidating self-definition and making basic connections between thoughts, feelings, and emotions. This occurs for those just emerging from the Surviving Phase as well as those starting to revert into the Surviving Phase. Others in the Existing Phase display a better defined sense of self and greater metacognitive capacity, but remain restricted emotionally, interpersonally, and behaviorally. These individuals exhibit greater readiness and receptivity to more exploratory therapies. Those experiencing a first-episode psychosis or a briefer, less developed psychosis may recover more quickly to this level of functioning and, thereby, more readily engage in and respond to interventions of greater depth and breadth. In the program at a state psychiatric hospital in the United States, to further differentiate those within the Existing Phase and better tailor services, individuals with characteristics nearer to the Surviving Phase were informally referred to as "Existing- (minus)" and those beginning to approximate the Living Phase were considered "Existing+ (plus)." These modifications highlight that the model continues to be shaped as clinicians respond to the varied presentations of persons experiencing psychosis.

Unique characteristics of care in the Existing Phase

Once the individual is more assured of his existence and safety and begins to display a more consistent, coherent self, the therapist gradually can incorporate more typical ways of engaging and intervening with the client. Interactions will begin to be more like waves over a rock rather than over sand and the therapy relationship can be experienced as a joint interaction that fortifies the self rather than overtakes it. Specifically, the individual becomes more receptive and responsive to the therapeutic interventions described recently to address psychosis, such as with increasing opportunities to explore thoughts and feelings, utilization of the therapy relationship, skill building, and exploring meaning and the historical antecedents of hallucinations and delusions (Alanen, 1997; Hingley, 2006; Kingdon and Turkington, 2005). For example, cognitive-behavioral therapies (CBT) recently have re-established the role of psychotherapy in the treatment of the psychoses, including for those diagnosed with schizophrenia, particularly with individuals who are willing to actively participate in treatment and display "at least minimal insight into the abnormal nature of their experiences" (Silverstein et al., 2006). Additionally, the initial steps described by Semerari et al. (2003) for developing the self-reflectivity aspect of metacognition can be introduced once there is at least a minimal ability to examine the self. Enhancing metacognitive abilities, or one's ability to think about thinking, is fundamental to interventions targeting thoughts and feelings, as well as for improving functional outcome (Koren et al., 2006). More exploratory interventions, related to thoughts, feelings, and interpersonal experiences, can prove useful once an implicit sense of existence is established and the individual is able to at least minimally interact with another and reflect on the self as a thinking being. Clients in the Existing Phase, with emerging awareness of self and other, are more likely to participate and to display such capabilities.

As such, CBT strategies can be effectively integrated into a psychodynamic framework that continuously assesses the status of the individual, including the level of self-definition, awareness of others, and capacity to recognize thoughts and feelings, in guiding the type and timing of interventions. In particular, fluctuations in self-experience, along with changes in emotional and cognitive functioning, even within a single session, necessitate frequent adjustments by the therapist to tailor interventions. For example, the therapist may shift from exploration of thoughts and feelings back to supportive reassurance of safety and self-defining work if the client becomes more distressed, threatened, disorganized and less self-aware. In this way, the therapist continuously modifies the nature and level of interaction between therapist and client in order to maintain an effective therapeutic encounter.

During this phase, the focus of therapy turns to helping the client further define himself as well as to increase awareness of others, to begin to explore the meaning of psychotic responses, to increase awareness of thoughts and feelings, and to teach alternative, reality-based means of coping. The duration of a therapy session is likely closer to the standard fifty-minute length and there may be both a present and future focus. The remainder of this chapter will describe specific aspects to psychological interventions for individuals during the Existing Phase.

Treatment strategies for the Existing Phase

Continue to promote differentiation and sense of self

As discussed in detail in the previous chapter, schizophrenia has been described as fundamentally a disorder of the self that necessitates the goal of developing a sense of a coherent self in the client (Pollack, 1989). Interventions in the Existing Phase, therefore, continue to target fortifying the person as a separate individual and enhancing identity and self-confidence, as bolstering self-concept and self-esteem has been found to be important in recovery from a psychotic episode (Roe, 2003). As differentiation progresses, identification with others needs to be counterbalanced with enhancing self-definition in order to continue to fend off concerns about merger.

As an example, from the beginning of treatment, a man diagnosed with paranoid schizophrenia had frequently mentioned a book he enjoyed. He initially became anxious and declined to describe anything that he liked about the book but, as he began to view himself as more of a separate individual (i.e., his self was emerging and becoming defined) and was frequently reassured that he was a different person from the therapist, he was able to talk more about the story and read aloud a few passages to the therapist. Approximately six months into the therapy, the therapist informed him that she had decided to read the book, thinking that it must be interesting if he had enjoyed it so much. It was thought that informing the client of this would add to his sense of being a separate person with valued ideas and opinions. However, the client immediately became anxious, started thumbing through the book and saying "I don't know what you will think" and "there may be a few bad parts in here," clearly worrying about what the book might say about him. The therapist said, "We will probably discover that you and I may respond to some things in this book differently and other things similarly. That is what will be interesting. But, you know, the person this book is going to tell me the most about is Jack London, because he wrote it." The client looked up with enormous relief and said, "Really? I guess that's right." Discussion continued about the book reflecting the author and also that readers have some similar and different reactions. A few sessions later, the client asked what the therapist thought of the book and engaged in a lively discussion about it without the prior level of anxiety and agitation that comes with fearing one is being found out and engulfed. He also stated, "It means a lot to me that you wanted to read a book I had read. No one has ever done that before." He could not have experienced being valued until he was differentiated from the therapist and from the book.

The previous example also highlights the continued importance of exploring and fostering the individual's interests, preferences, needs, and aspirations to further enhance self-definition. The individual's goals for recovery may be further elicited and articulated in this phase as the guidepost for treatment planning. As the individual is emerging from the storm and/or shelter of psychosis, multidisciplinary efforts to encourage activities and interactions contribute to this goal in ways that reawaken, reassure, and reconnect the individual. In addition to psychotherapy, many other professional and peer professional services, including recreational therapy outings, occupational therapy sensory awareness interventions, and vocational therapy, promote self-definition and development.

Basic self-structure requires connection between the physical and psychological self as separate, but related, aspects. That is, as the individual starts to feel a return of the "soul" (as many describe), a re-acquaintance and reconnection with the body, and with thoughts and feelings, is necessary. This process is sometimes manifested in hyper-focus on the body and what is wrong with it or, conversely, in ignoring and avoiding focus on the body. An overly somatic focus for the individual can occur to an extent that the physical concerns consume and define the person rather than be experienced as one aspect of the person's experience. Whereas in the Surviving Phase, the somatic hyper-focus may result in somatic delusions reflecting such concerns as disintegration (e.g., "my organs are falling apart") or distorted threat perceptions ("Satan is in my penis"), somatic preoccupations in the Existing Phase may be distorted, but to a lesser extent, and reflect efforts to define the self in relation to the body. One related goal, then, is to facilitate awareness of bodily experiences as one aspect of the self rather than the whole self, such as by providing education about how physical sensations provide information (emotional or physical), identifying parts of the body that feel okay (i.e., are not causing pain or concern), and facilitating recognition that physical symptoms may reflect emotional experiences. For those individuals who move from complete lack of awareness and/or denial of the physical self in the Surviving Phase to the Existing Phase, continued efforts to help the person be aware of the body, physical characteristics, and basic self-care are remedial.

Increase awareness of others

As the person begins to feel more connected within himself (between body and mind), the emphasis shifts more to a connection with others. Within the therapy relationship, this emerging awareness of others results in transference issues becoming clearer and provides useful information to the therapist. However, the client in the Existing Phase generally is not ready for extensive exploration of the source of the transference or interpretations, but is in need of respectful, often corrective, interpersonal experiences. It is important to demonstrate with actions a trusting, respectful, and egalitarian approach, but also to articulate the nature of the relationship in words to make these characteristics explicit for the client. Making it explicit helps to increase the sense of safety as well as to immediately indicate that the clinician differs from expectations and past negative experiences. That is, the focus remains primarily on accurate appraisal of the present relationship and remedial experiences. For example, if a client expresses that people are always trying to control him, the response might be, "That is not my goal. The purpose of therapy is for you to continue to increase control over your own life and experiences. If you want, our meetings can be to assist you in that." As another example, a client stated, "You always start by asking me the same questions each time and I don't know what to say." He expressed feeling pressured each time to come up with topics of discussion when asked how he was doing or what he would like to talk about that day. He offered that this recapitulated an early childhood experience of feeling inadequate, fearful of being "stupid," and potentially shamed. The connection between his concerns about therapy and early childhood experiences was not explored further at that time, given his vulnerability to psychotic regression when emotionally pressed. Instead, he was thanked for expressing his concern and was engaged in problem-solving ways to make it more comfortable to start the session. In this way, he was engaged as an equal partner in the therapy rather than as a passive victim.

Another way to assist in increasing accurate appraisal (and, thereby, lessen the sense of threat) within the therapy relationship is to request specific examples when a client begins to include the therapist in paranoid projections. For example, when a client says "You guys ..." followed by some perception of persecution, threat, or punishment, the therapist can comment, "I am not 'you guys,' I am just one person. Is there something in particular that I have said or done that has you thinking that I am out to get you?" Such an intervention shifts the client's appraisal from being based on general expectations or fears of unknown or unseen others to the immediate, specific experience of the therapeutic relationship.

Another, more complicated example underscores that, particularly with a paranoid individual, intentions are made explicit, but not necessarily the therapist's feelings toward the person. A man who consistently thwarted efforts for others to care about him, told his therapist of many years that no one would care if he died. The therapist stated, "I get paid to see and help people, but I don't get paid to have them matter to me. That is up to me." The therapist's caring was expressed in this rather elusive, almost indifferent, manner to match the client's more distant stance in order to assist him in tolerating it. He would not have been able to tolerate the therapist directly stating that she cared about him. In response, the client laughed derisively and expressed that he sometimes felt "condescended to in here." The therapist paused and then replied, "I am thinking about what you said about feeling condescended to. I can understand that and I am sorry if you have felt that way in here. That is certainly not my intention. It is not okay for others to treat you that way and you, also, do enough condescending of yourself (*client nods and laughs*)." After a pause, he responded, "maybe I just try to make myself unlovable." In this situation, the therapist was explicit about not trying to condescend to him, and then that projection (which was his tendency to look down upon himself and others) was returned to him. Such interventions highlight that clearly verbalizing expectations and experiences in the therapy relationship is important for facilitating accurate appraisal, enhancing safety, and reducing the distortions that might confirm a client's negative expectations and recapitulate past experiences.

In summary, the emerging awareness of self-being-with-other creates opportunities for the topic of the therapy relationship itself to be carefully broached and more positive relational experiences to occur. In addition, as the individual experiences a clearer boundary between self and other, judicious use of therapist self-disclosure for the purpose of normalizing may be more appropriate and effective than in the Surviving Phase. This might include descriptions of mutual innocuous interests, activities, or emotional experiences that validate the client. Concerns about other relationships become a focus of therapy in the Existing Phase as well, providing opportunities to normalize, educate, and assist the client in dealing more effectively interpersonally. The importance of specific social skills training is elaborated later in this chapter.

Continue family work

An important part of self–other work in the Existing Phase involves continuing to explore and address family relationships and the effect on the client. Family issues can be problem-solved within individual sessions as well as, when appropriate, in structured family therapy sessions. Inclusion of family in therapy generally is very important if the individual lives with them; however, it may be contraindicated if the individual lives independent of family. When deemed appropriate, family sessions may start via telephone and gradually move toward Internet or live family sessions, depending upon the individual's level of stress tolerance. The therapist ensures that family sessions provide in vivo practice in having a specific focus to discussions, in communication and problem-solving that is calm and effective without high expressed emotion, and in respecting individual strengths and differences. Individual sessions can address current concerns and problem-solve and role-play in preparation for interactions with family. In addition, exploration of the person's perceptions of family relationships in individual therapy not only elucidates past and current concerns contributing to difficulties, but also portends of expectations in current relationships, including with the therapist.

For example, a man who described his mother as controlling, self-serving, and untrustworthy readily perceived the therapist as intrusive and untrustworthy. Further, his struggle with whether his mother's attentions were inappropriate ("I think my mother is in love with me") were repeated in his tendency to sexualize the therapy relationship. In this situation, in addition to maintaining and discussing clear boundaries within the therapy relationship, the therapist set limits on the frequent calls that the man's mother made to the therapist. This modeled limit setting for the client. It also reduced the tendency to merge the therapist and mother in the client's perceptions. Both the client and the mother were encouraged in developing alternative supports as part of reducing their interdependency. Family sessions were not conducted, given the goal of fostering independence, but considerable focus was spent in individual sessions on family-related issues. A brief session was conducted, however, with this same man and his father, when his father visited him at the hospital. In sessions prior to the visit, the client expressed significant fears about his father, past negative experiences, as well as concern for the therapist in meeting him. The family session afforded opportunity to validate the father's concerns and engage him in his son's goals, while highlighting his son's independence and strengths. The therapist was able to model for the client how to help his father manage his temper (which he had lost with another staff member the same day) such as by the comment "I can see that you feel strongly about your son's treatment and I want to hear what you have to say. However, I will be able to hear you better if you can lower your voice." The two were encouraged to spend time doing something enjoyable the remainder of the day, which they were able to do. The brief family session empowered the client with hope as well as some strategies for future interactions with his father.

Overall, family work in the Existing Phase continues to promote differentiation, while beginning to explore family relationships and address related issues. Past experiences and current concerns are addressed and efforts are made to begin to define the role the individual wants to play within the family system. Provision of support to an involved family is important as well. The different forms of family therapy work, including psychodynamic, behavioral, and systemic, can be tailored to the needs and capabilities of the individual during the Existing Phase. More detailed accounts of family therapy interventions can be found elsewhere (e.g., Thorsen *et al.*, 2006).

Increase awareness of and influence over thought processes

As previously noted, as the client develops increasing awareness of his or her thoughts as a separate but important part of the self (i.e., s/he displays the metacognitive ability to examine cognitions), the person may be more responsive to interventions that target thought processes. This includes elements of cognitive behavior therapies. Only some examples of interventions pertaining to thinking are described here: The reader is referred to more comprehensive sources for detailed descriptions of CBT for psychosis (e.g., Beck *et al.*, 2009; Hagen *et al.*, 2011; Kingdon, and Turkington, 2005). Any interventions that target thought processes in the Existing Phase start with assessing and strengthening the extent to which the individual possesses adequate awareness of personal thoughts, can distinguish thoughts from actions, understands that automatic thoughts are normal, and can monitor thoughts. These represent prerequisites for more advanced interventions, such as increasing mental flexibility, altering attributions, and learning information processing strategies. For those transitioning from the Surviving Phase, awareness of thinking may be very basic initially. A client realized one day, "I can have a thought and have it all day." Another expressed, "The thing that ticks me off [i.e., angers me] the most is not being able to hold on to a thought for more than a second for the past six years. It's the thievery." Another man asked, "Is worrying the same as thinking?" Consistent with the Surviving Phase, the therapist can continue to point out when a client is having a thought, normalize, and distinguish thoughts from feelings and from actions.

As fundamental thinking processes are evident, additional strategies can be introduced. For example, improving accuracy in the cognitive appraisal of experiences, including within the therapy relationship as described earlier in the chapter, is another aspect of cognitive interventions in the Existing Phase. Aspects to this strategy include seeking facts to support an assumption and generating alternative explanations in order to enhance belief flexibility and to reduce the tendency to jump to conclusions (Kingdon and Turkington, 2005). It also involves assessing situations based on the present information rather than past experiences. For example, upon hearing the sound of a drill next door to the therapy room, one client immediately began to express concern that people were trying to drill into her head. She was quickly placated when informed of the construction work being done and reassured that no one would be entering the therapy room. In another situation, a male client appeared alarmed to see his therapist at the grocery store when he was working there. In the subsequent session, when asked how it was to see his therapist at his workplace, the client expressed feeling like she had been checking up on him. The fact that the therapist regularly shopped there and that, coincidentally, he was working when she went, was discussed. His initial statement of "feeling like" she had been checking on him was a sign of progress in that it indicated that he did not believe with certainty his explanation of her reason for being there, that it only felt that way. In a more regressed state of the Surviving Phase, a more paranoid individual would believe with conviction that he was being checked up on at work and would not have exhibited the cognitive flexibility that this man did.

As another example, regarding command hallucinations, a benign cognitive challenge is to ask the individual what s/he would do in a given hypothetical situation, such as if the therapist told him to jump in the lake.

Client:	I wouldn't do it.
Therapist:	Why not?
Client:	Because I don't want to.
Therapist:	What will happen if you don't do it?
Client:	Nothing.
Therapist:	That's right. I can't make you do anything and nothing would happen if you chose not to do it. You are in charge of yourself and can decide whether you do what I or others say, or believe what I or others say. It's the same thing with voices. You may not be able to decide if they occur, but you can decide if you listen to them, just like you can with people in your life.

This discussion not only challenges beliefs about the omnipotence of voices, but also further empowers and reassures the client of individuality and interpersonal choices, including in the therapy.

A part of the above example echoes therapy interventions made in the 1980s emphasizing that a person cannot control hearing voices, but can decide whether to believe the voices and whether to try to understand the meaning behind the experience (Karon and Vandenbos, 1981). This understanding, that altering the perception of distressing voices is an important part of therapy, has been continued and expanded upon in current CBT approaches. Such interventions are an important part of work in the Existing Phase and are based on the premise that a person's attributions about voices influence his reactions to the voice-hearing experience. In particular, the more the individual perceives voices to be real, threatening, and influential, the more distressed he will be in response to the experience. A teenager, for example, was highly distressed by command hallucinations telling him to look directly into the sun. The therapist inquired, "What will happen if you don't do what the voices say?" After a long pause, the client indicated that he didn't know. It was then discussed how long he had been hearing the voices (months) without acting upon what they were commanding him to do and without any consequence. Recognizing that he had already been able to listen to his own voice telling him not to look in the sun without penalty lowered his distress. Similarly, as the individual is able to attribute voice-hearing to his level of present stress or to being reminded of experiences of the past, distress related to the experience diminishes.

As fundamental thinking processes are honed, cognitive remediation techniques, such as teaching information processing strategies, can also be conducted. However, that the techniques are sometimes taught using guided mental imagery highlights the necessity of first ensuring sufficient metacognitive capacity to participate. A variant of cognitive therapy interventions is Acceptance and Commitment Therapy or ACT (Hayes *et al.*, 1999). Similar to other cognitive interventions for psychosis, ACT facilitates awareness of thoughts (including regarding hallucinations and delusions), but the goal is to acknowledge the thoughts without trying to avoid or dispute them. Session exercises provide opportunities to practice mindfulness with psychotic symptoms, noting thoughts and perceptions without attaching meaning, acting on the thoughts, or believing them. Ford (2005) describes mindfulness as part of a cognitive process for improving the ability to discriminate between relevant and irrelevant information and suggests that interventions emphasize eliciting and reinforcing accurate perceptions rather than disputing distorted beliefs and experiences. These strategies underscore the importance of acknowledgment of hallucinations and delusions in order to progress, which runs contrary to the tendency of individuals with severe psychosis to deny or suppress the experiences. Denial initially is due to a lack of alternative means of coping; however, during treatment, clients also quickly learn to deny symptoms to treatment professionals due to (often substantiated) fears of prolonged hospitalization or being given additional psychotropic medications. As one experienced psychiatrist noted, "Patients often are discharged when they stop *saying* they are hearing voices, not when they stop experiencing them." Treatment goals, then, need to include increasing awareness that directly acknowledging distressing voices and beliefs can be managed and can be more beneficial than avoidance and denial.

Begin to make meaning of hallucinations

Both psychodynamic therapies and CBT emphasize thorough assessment of factors involved in the development and maintenance of hallucinations and delusions for conceptualizing and intervening. Hallucinations can be understood as reflecting internal experiences, impulses, or memories that have been falsely attributed to sources outside of the self. Delusions represent efforts to explain experiences and, often, to compensate for unmet needs. The goal of interventions is to gradually accept hallucinations and delusions as one's own in a more realistic and manageable way and develop more adaptive ways to express and to address issues. It is important to note, however, that these interventions not only require metacognitive abilities, but also the psychological readiness to accept what were previously intolerable thoughts, experiences, and impulses. During the Existing Phase, when the client is no longer in acute crisis, therapy can focus more on assessing the development of the individual's psychotic responses and to make meaning of psychotic symptoms, both as responses to stress and as ways to protect the self from perceived threats. The client may begin to examine some of the stressors (past and present) that contribute to his difficulties, although exploration of more emotionally provoking memories, particularly traumatic ones, must be carefully titrated and paced based on the individual's level of tolerance for stress.

As mentioned in Chapter 2, a particular challenge that arises in therapy is to find a way to explore delusional content and hallucinations without colluding with the experiences. This can be accomplished by keeping questions focused on details of the client's experience and reflecting on the themes, the related emotions, and what it provides for the individual. At times, it is important to acknowledge that "you and I may see this differently, and I just want to understand more about how you see it." This introduces the client to the idea that there is more than one way to perceive his/her experience.

Eliciting specific details about the current voice-hearing experience, which may have started in the Surviving Phase, continues in the Existing Phase. Information to obtain about auditory hallucinations includes the number of voices heard, their gender and ages, the content of the speech, and whether the speech includes commands. It also is important to determine which voices are perceived to be pleasant, neutral, or distressing, the degree of perceived influence over the individual, as well as what intensifies or lessens their intrusion upon the individual. It takes careful and intentional effort by the therapist to conduct this exploration in such a way that it conveys interest and collaboration, rather than intrusion. As details about the current experience are understood, the client and therapist begin to examine the initial development of the hallucinations. Often, when asked, the individual can readily provide the time at which s/he first started hearing voices. The client also may be asked whether the voices remind them of anyone in her life. Delineating the context in which the voices were first heard often provides critical information about the voices' meaning and purpose. Hallucinations may reflect and/or defend against many themes, including traumatic memories, feelings of rage, fears for safety, or needs for companionship. Some hallucinations may be seen as a distorted re-experiencing of past trauma (Read and Ross, 2003). The origin and meaning of the hallucinations can be discovered within the therapy relationship, sometimes formulating rapidly and, other times, unfolding slowly over time as fragments are woven together.

Begin to make meaning of delusions

Assessment of the specifics of a belief deemed to be delusional also continues in the Existing Phase. In addition to obtaining specifics about the belief, it is also important to assess the extent to which the person believes a particular notion to be true. The answers indicate the amount of cognitive flexibility versus rigidity that exists at the outset of therapy. The question can be posed as: "If you could give a percentage, how certain are you that this is true?" This converts the belief from a bifurcated true or false conviction to an idea whose degree of veracity lies on a continuum. The question also is phrased in a positive manner in order to reduce defensiveness.

In one case, a woman adamantly insisted that her former boss came to visit her at her group home and had sexual relations with her there. Because she had 24-hour supervision, it was considered unlikely that this was occurring. In addition, she previously had described having an affair with a different man who would visit her apartment. She had 24-hour supervision in that placement as well and, when asked to describe sexual relations, her responses indicated a lack of knowledge of sexual activity, including about sexual intercourse. However, the more her family, staff, and other treatment professionals challenged her about the truth of her experience, the more rigidly she adhered to her conviction that it was true. In therapy, she was supported in how much she wanted to have a relationship and how good it can feel to be attractive to someone as well as to be in love. Within this more supportive context, when asked the percentage question by her therapist, she paused and then estimated "about 80 percent." While she was not ready at that time to explore the reasons why she might not fully believe it to be true, she had allowed herself and the therapist to recognize that there was some doubt in her mind. As supportive others stopped challenging her regarding her beliefs, and interventions focused on improving her present relationships and increasing opportunities to meet others, she eventually noted in therapy that she hadn't seen her lover for some time and he "seemed to be moving on," and added, "I need to do so as well." While her erotomanic delusion would be classified as a "nonbizarre" delusion, it significantly interfered with her functioning in that it resulted in extensive withdrawal into a fantasy world involving the relationship. It also impaired her work and her relationships. Her resolution to her belief, that he had moved on and that she needed to do so as well, allowed her to preserve her self-esteem. It also provided opportunity to explore feelings of rejection, inadequacy, and longing for a relationship.

After eliciting information about the specifics of the belief and the extent of the belief, exploration of how it developed is an important collaborative journey for the client and therapist. This is both assessment and intervention in addressing delusional beliefs. Merely inquiring about when the individual began to understand or believe the idea implies that it has not always been true or evident. Identifying the context in which a belief developed also leads to insight and understanding about the origin of the belief, creating a foundation for formulating factors that contributed to the development of the belief and identifying purposes the belief may serve.

Different types of delusions can reflect recapitulation of unresolved issues or traumatic events, project unwanted memories, feelings, or thoughts, attempt to compensate for intense feelings of inadequacy, or provide companionship. Sometimes even the most seemingly incredible expressed beliefs may have some vestige of truth in them. One man on an inpatient psychiatric unit continued to talk about a "Dr. Jones" (a fictitious name) within seemingly nonsensical, rapid verbalizations. Although difficult to understand, there appeared to be worries in the extended verbalizations about Dr. Jones' death and the client's contribution to it. However, the entire content was considered by most staff to be illogical gibberish. However, inquiry into the hospital history revealed that the individual had been a patient during the time, decades prior, when a Dr. Jones was working at the hospital. When the patient was asked about what happened, he indicated that he had told the psychiatrist his story "and later that night he killed himself." The psychiatrist had, indeed, killed himself and his wife during the time that the patient was at the hospital. When he was informed by his therapist that the doctor had had serious problems and that it was not his fault that the man died, he appeared extremely relieved and stated, "I have always thought it was my fault." For over thirty years he had been tormented by guilt over a misperceived traumatic event. Although this situation is a more extreme example, it underscores the caution needed to not immediately discount the content of what a person says.

When factual basis cannot be found to support a belief, the themes still convey important information about issues with which the person is struggling, underscoring the importance of understanding the meaning and purpose of the delusion. For example, grandiose delusions may compensate for perceived inadequacies, such as the man who had been discharged from the military for mental health reasons who would talk about currently being an active duty, 5-star general or the inpatient, destitute male who would talk about having millions of dollars. Referential delusions, in which the person perceives information (such as from media, songs, or comments or gestures from others) to be specifically about him, can reflect grandiosity, feelings of intrusion, and/or paranoia and persecution. Paranoid, persecutory delusions are very common in those diagnosed with schizophrenia and may reflect grandiosity (one has to be quite important to have the FBI after them) as well as fears of interpersonal harm, which are often founded in past interpersonal victimizations. Somatic delusions involve experiences of the body, such as being invaded in some way (objects in the penis or rectum), disintegration of body parts, infestation with bugs, or emitting a foul odor. These reflect fears of onslaught and/or invasion of the body, which may have roots in prior physical or sexual abuse or other experiences of interpersonal victimization. Somatic delusions of disintegration tend to emerge when a person is particularly regressed and poignantly express the experience of "falling apart." Somatic delusions pose challenges to clinicians in determining what may be an actual medical concern, a distortion of an existing medical problem, or an experience without medical basis. More often there may elements of truth in the event or the perceptions or feelings that the individual has that warrant attention, support, and understanding and it is the therapist's task to listen to the content of the delusion and determine if there is some vestige of a true characteristic or concern of the individual.

One man developed delusional beliefs to explain his experience of auditory hallucinations. He was convinced that his voices were caused by some unidentified, malevolent individual manipulating his thoughts by interfering with sound frequencies. He researched the possibilities extensively on the internet and wrote articulate, well-organized letters to several government agencies. His hope was to find a more palatable, externalized explanation for his difficulties as an alternative to just being "sick" and "crazy." It was particularly difficult to explore alternative explanations for his problems to these two options (i.e., that either someone out there was doing this to him or he was just crazy) because the majority of his health care system emphasized that his "symptoms" were just his mental illness. It was progress that he was able to acknowledge hearing voices and having some problems, but his belief in the cause highlighted his feelings of victimization, his avoidance of introspection (i.e., of focusing at all on himself, his own thoughts and feelings, and the effect on his experience), and his external locus of control. The beliefs were also grandiose in nature as a means to compensate for the terrible onslaught to his self-esteem that his prolonged hospitalization and impairing problems were to him. The theme in the delusions of someone intentionally harming him also was consistent with the emotional and physical abuse he had endured as a child.

Explore alternatives to hallucinations and delusions

As the purposes of problematic beliefs and hallucinations are identified, the individual begins to have greater insight into the problems created by such perceptions. As one man said, "I think I have problems in thinking and you think so, too." The therapist gradually increases awareness of the disadvantages of continuing to rely on such means of coping while, concurrently, strengthening alternative means of dealing with the issues. The individual may be receptive to exploring ways in which the belief interferes with his life and his goals and negative aspects may be collaboratively identified. Alternative explanations and supportive evidence for problematic beliefs, well described in cognitive interventions for delusions (e.g., Kingdon and Turkington, 2005), may be investigated together. Generally, confirming and contradictory evidence of a strongly held belief are discussed gradually and gently in order to work collaboratively and to avoid defensive reactions that result in fortifying a position. As with any type of intervention, cognitive interventions are more likely to be effective with recently developed problematic ideas than those that have persisted for many years.

Additional intervention strategies include normalization and validation of what are perceived to be unaccepted thoughts, feelings, or impulses, with efforts to acknowledge them and reintegrate them into the person's internal experience. Teaching more adaptive ways to express emotions, drawing out the individual's strengths, and facilitating participation in activities that bolster self-esteem and develop satisfying social interactions also are included. Psycho-education about effects of trauma and, eventually, emotionally processing past events, is often a part of intervention. These interventions occur as direct and adjunctive services in treatment, with the goal that, as more adaptive means address the issues underlying the delusion or hallucination, they will not be needed as much. There will be a gradual loosening and letting go of the belief and reductions in the distress related to hallucinations. For example, that delusions frequently reflect efforts to compensate for and defend against feelings of inadequacy necessitates gradually assisting the client in becoming aware of the feelings and experiences that underlie the delusion. This will only be possible, however, if the individual has adequate alternative sources bolstering the sense of adequacy and ability to tolerate those emotions more directly and effectively. The individual who states that he is a CEO of a Fortune 500 company will only be able to relinquish the beliefs as he begins to experience self-worth in reality-based experiences and relationships. He also needs to have the psychological resources to tolerate, initially in a mitigated, manageable manner, a sense that he feels that he has not "measured up." In response to such grandiose delusions, the therapist might respond, "Well, even if you weren't those things, you and I know that you are a valuable person who is worthwhile" and subsequently identify reality-based attributes or accomplishments of the person.

To illustrate, when exploring with a man who described possessing a special line through which he communicated in thought with others (a sort of two-way brain radio), it was discovered that it originally developed within the context of significant sibling rivalry, the loss of his job, and distressing marital difficulties, including an alleged affair by his wife. During these intense, multiple stressors, he began to believe he was visited and appointed by God with special abilities and he began to believe that his children and his wife were satanic. His subsequent actions frightened and distanced his family from him and he was hospitalized. He subsequently developed an elaborate delusional system in which he would connect to a line that kept him connected to his family as well as to famous individuals. His delusional system defended against grief, loneliness, guilt, and feelings of inadequacy. When exploring the potential purpose of his special line, he stated, "If I don't have it, I don't have anything. I will be totally alone and have to accept that I live at the hospital and don't have a life." To protect himself from the intense affect related to this realization, he immediately began talking about being a god and not a human being. Therapy for him focused on continuing to increase his ability to tolerate some of the emotions and cognitions he was working to defend against, such as acknowledgment that his problems and behavior had resulted in estrangement from loved ones. Therapy also explored the accompanying grief and anger at himself, while also trying to foster his strengths, interests, activities, and current social support to offset his losses, bolster self-esteem, and provide incentive to focus on his current, reality-based life. He would not be able to relinquish his delusions involving the special line of communication until he developed other means to manage his intense emotions, painful memories, and negative self-perceptions. Just as the rehabilitation specialist would not take crutches from someone before the person had either something else to lean on or stronger legs, the psychotherapist must not work to "take away" a person's delusion, but help the person develop healthier, effective alternatives. As this occurs, reliance on a delusion can diminish. In this case, although the client talked about "getting off of" his special line, which put considerable pressure upon him, the therapist encouraged him just to allow it to be there, but also to expand his options.

Begin to assess for possible dissociative experiences

Given the significant overlap between positive symptoms of psychosis and dissociation, the high prevalence of dissociative symptoms in individuals diagnosed with schizophrenia, and the high rates of trauma in the histories of individuals with severe forms of psychosis, it is important to begin to evaluate for dissociative symptoms when the person is in the Existing Phase. These symptoms include cognitive lapses, emotional numbing, feelings of derealization, and altered body experiences. Assessment of such symptoms can be challenging because the individual may have limited insight and may be reluctant or yet unable to do the introspection and discussion of internal experiences required. Nonetheless, the Existing Phase can be a time for the mental health clinician to start assessing and further raising the person's awareness of his/her experiences and ways of responding. For example, just noting when the person seems distracted during a discussion ("It seems you went away for minute. Where did you go? Did something distract you?") invites the individual to start to observe his/her experience. More extensive assessment and intervention can occur in the Living Phase, as described in Chapter 4, and more information regarding the overlap between dissociation and psychosis is provided in Chapter 5.

Increase affective awareness and improve emotion regulation

Given the critical roles that affectivity and stress play in relapses for those experiencing psychosis (Bebbington *et al.*, 1993), ongoing efforts in therapy to improve emotion regulation and coping are important in treatment of psychosis. This includes teaching emotion identification and adaptive emotional expression (Penn and Combs, 2000). The limited tolerance for affect in the Existing Phase, however, underscores the importance of limited and carefully planned use of emotional material (expressed by the therapist or the client). As one client noted, "I don't want to talk about my feelings, because then someone might steal them." Another client was uncomfortable with having felt angry. When the therapist normalized that he was experiencing emotions just as everyone does, he agreed but distanced himself by saying, "Yeah, I knew a guy once in the 70s at a 7-Eleven [store] who was in a bad mood." Given the tendency for significant denial and avoidance of emotion, then, one initial step is to introduce emotional experiences in a mitigated form within the context of normalizing the experience such as, "I don't know if this is true for you or not, but most people would be a bit bothered if someone locked them out of their own room." Such statements provide opportunity for the individual to agree or disagree and facilitate the individual gradually building the stamina for managing affective experience. Progress in emotional awareness and regulation is evident when the therapist is able to directly ask the person about a specific emotion, although generally still in a mitigated form. The therapist titrates up to inquiring about emotions in an unmitigated form, such as by asking if the client is angry at a particular person or attracted to a certain person. All the discussions need to continue to be introduced within the context of normalizing the experiences as well as emphasizing the individual's ability to manage the emotions surfacing into awareness.

A man whose escalating paranoia resulted in threatening neighbors and the police was subsequently incarcerated and then hospitalized on a forensic unit for many years. He was able to reconstitute within the structure and support of an inpatient unit and medications to lower his arousal and distress. As he progressed to the Existing Phase and was transferred to a residential, outpatient unit, he displayed more "I" statements and was clearer in his self-definition. He managed adequately by working minimal hours at a hospital job and by maintaining a routine. He denied interest in developing hobbies or participating in enjoyable activities, noting that he preferred to "keep it simple." As he progressed, preparations were made for him to move from a hospital-based apartment to an apartment in the community. Although he initially expressed looking forward to moving off-campus, when the move was delayed due to lack of availability, he was reluctant to acknowledge his frustration and stress. He denied these feelings, noting that he equated any "negative" emotion with having severe problems and feared his emotions might get out of hand, and that he might "get crazy." At the start of a therapy session during this time period, he became agitated and started to talk about how he was the doctor, and how he had been the jailer when in jail. Such illogical statements reflected the more diffuse boundaries he was experiencing between self and other (specifically, the therapist) under stress. Because he generally had been displaying stronger psychological resources, he was directly asked how he was feeling about the delay in his move. Although he minimized his feelings about it, he immediately became less anxious and more focused when the topic was introduced. After his frustration and stress about the delay as well as about moving were normalized, he resumed talking logically and with better self-definition (i.e., without statements confusing his role with others). In this case, the cause of his distress was directly addressed in order to reduce his anxiety and return him to reality-based coping. If he had not responded to this intervention, the therapist would have returned to more supportive, self-defining interventions to facilitate reconstitution from his lapse into the Surviving Phase. He subsequently was encouraged to continue to acknowledge and directly express feelings about his move.

As the individual responds to these initial interventions, other emotion regulation strategies may be introduced and practiced. Strategies may include Dialectical Behavior Therapy techniques found beneficial with other trauma-related disorders (Dimeff and Linehan, 2001), such as acknowledgment and acceptance of emotions without judging (e.g., "I am nervous about going to a new group") and mindfulness techniques. Identifying and employing strategies that reduce the intensity of an emotion, such as mental and behavioral distractions and relaxation skills, may also be developed.

Provide psycho-education and teach adaptive coping skills

The increasing awareness of self and others generally renders individuals in the Existing Phase more receptive to psycho-education about coping and social skills as well as about factors that may have contributed to development of psychotic symptoms. For example, CBT emphasizes normalizing psychotic experiences (Pfammatter *et al.*, 2006), such as by discussing famous individuals who have experienced visual or auditory hallucinations and discussing the role of stress and traumatic experiences in the development of psychotic symptoms. The stress-vulnerability model (Zubin and Spring, 1977) and early sensory deprivation studies are often described as a way of highlighting the role of stress and vulnerability factors. These discussions lay the groundwork for exploration of the specific factors and experiences that may have contributed to the development of an individual's particular psychotic responses.

Learning basic stress management skills is particularly important, not only because psychotic symptoms often occur during periods of anxiety or stress, but also because individuals often fear becoming acutely psychotic again, which contributes to restricting their experiences in an effort to reduce the risk of relapse (Shaw *et al.*, 2002). Simply being able to identify stressors and realizing/acknowledging that events can have an effect on a person may take some time. Daily issues related to social interactions, family, treatment, and work provide opportunities to problem-solve with a client. Given that individuals often remain sensitive to boundary intrusions in this phase, such informational efforts often remain better received when discussed more generally or offhandedly rather than directly about the client (e.g., "Many people feel less comfortable in a crowd"). The standard interventions that include the functional purposes of stress, exploring the physical responses, identifying personal warning signs of increasing stress, and specific stress reduction strategies also can be effective during this phase. Developing a 1 to 10 rating scale of the individual's stress level (1 = calm; 10 = very upset, stressed) is a useful practice for self-monitoring and provides a concrete, quantitative means of expressing one's experience.

As part of the growing awareness of others, there are opportunities to provide the basic social skills training frequently described, such as the use of didactic instruction, role-playing, and homework practice (Silverstein *et al.*, 2006). The fundamentals include learning the basic skills of assertiveness, such as leaving uncomfortable situations and saying "no" to others, as well as basic conversation skills and reducing behaviors that keep others away (e.g., talking with unseen others, yelling, and poor hygiene). However, one of the primary challenges in teaching assertiveness in the Existing Phase is that individuals in this phase often continue to deny feelings of anger. This denial results in reluctance to be assertive in order to avoid activating angry and aggressive feelings. Extended discussions about the differences between assertiveness and aggression are important, but a person likely will only believe there is a difference as s/he experiences it. That is, as the individual asserts his or her opinion and discovers that s/he does not get out of control *and* the recipient does not retaliate, the person may begin to understand a difference between aggression and assertiveness. Social skills training has been shown to improve social and personal functioning, reduce symptoms, and hospital recidivism (Pfammatter *et al.*, 2006).

Additionally, learning strategies for reducing social anxiety, such as graded exposure and relaxation techniques, is relevant to many individuals with psychosis. Stress and anxiety are sometimes easier experiences for the client to acknowledge than hallucinations or disturbances in thinking and, therefore, an easier topic to engage in for therapy. In addition, social anxiety frequently arises as a problem in daily living, resulting in opportunities for the therapist and client to strategize solutions together with often prompt, effective results. One man, in considering whether to start volunteering at a community event, talked about how many people in town were "devils," gave examples of how he knew that, and implied that, therefore, many people were not to be trusted. When queried, he did not remember how nervous he initially had been when he first started attending a community center in town a year earlier. The therapist reminded him that he and his staff had planned ways for him to manage his nervousness, including taking bathroom breaks, stepping outside, and having an anti-anxiety medication along with him. He then was able to note how comfortable he is in that setting now. This past experience served as a good example of the normal anxiety ("nervousness") that a person may feel when trying something new. When he reverted to talking about people being devils, the therapist said, "Well, I don't know about that, but I do know that it is typical for a person to have some concerns when they meet new people and do something new." A discussion then ensued normalizing that he might have concerns about what others may think of him and how they will act toward him, the possibility of stigma, and allowing people the opportunity to earn his trust at the community event like he had at the community center. He was encouraged just to meet the volunteer coordinator and to gradually increase his involvement.

Another client, prior to starting her first college course, had strongly denied any concerns about starting college. However, she returned after the first class and reported that the students were making racist comments toward her (she is Caucasian in a predominantly Caucasian class) and that the teacher had called her a "Nazi" when she was out of the classroom in the bathroom. The therapist said, "You have worked so hard to get into college. It takes a lot of courage to go into a first class. Many people find it a little uncomfortable at first and wonder what others will think of them and where they will fit in." The client nodded. "What are you thinking of telling people when they ask about you, like where you live?" Immediate, specific problem-solving about how to answer personal questions followed. In these examples, challenges that arose from starting to expand their life experiences provided opportunities in therapy to normalize concerns as well as problem-solve ways to adaptively cope.

Finally, given the high rates of substance abuse for those who experience psychosis, psycho-education regarding substance abuse and motivational interviewing to enhance engagement in the process of maintaining sobriety frequently are important concurrent treatment interventions. This may be provided in individual as well as in group therapies.

Increase the range of life experiences

Individuals often wish to remain in the greater safety and predictability of a more restricted and, thereby, more manageable life. Part of the therapeutic task in the Existing Phase, then, is to assist in gradually broadening the perceived psychological and physical safety zone. One experience-based expert aptly and poignantly described the importance of establishing a "comfort zone" from which to "gently work outwards" as part of recovery, which he did by gradually increasing how far he went outside of his apartment into his community (Sparrowhawk, 2009). This facilitates expanding the physical safety zone, interactions with others, and involvement in activities while, simultaneously, increasing the stress tolerance to manage those experiences.

As previously mentioned, in addition to the efforts made through psychotherapy to increase emotional, behavioral, and interpersonal experiences, other disciplines assist clients in expanding other areas of their lives. Recreational therapists help clients increase leisure activities, vocational therapists assist in obtaining and maintaining a job, and occupational therapists and case managers promote independence in daily living, including with shopping, household care, self-care, and budgeting. Experience-based experts provide invaluable peer support and therapeutic assistance that facilitates expansion of the "comfort zone" and demonstrates the possibility of recovery. These important interventions develop essential life skills, bolster self-efficacy, and emphasize development of meaningful social roles and a sense of social inclusion, while supporting the client as s/he finds that increasing the range of life experiences can be done safely and satisfactorily. Staff or trusted others may accompany clients initially on new excursions and then gradually reduce direct support as the individual increases in comfort and competency. The longer the individual has been hospitalized, of course, the more difficult and crucial it is to reduce the dependency on the system and revive confidence in the individual's own capabilities.

Return projections

The client's ability to begin to acknowledge, tolerate, and manage his emotional reactions to contemporary situations serves as the foundation for starting to explore the purpose of projections, with the eventual goal of integrating those aspects into the self. That is, the goal is for the individual to eventually "own" his projections. As part of this, interpretations such as, "Your voices say some negative things about you that you also seem to think and believe at times," may be better received than by those in the Surviving Phase, but also depend on the individual's readiness and development of alternative means for coping. For example, in the second therapy session with a man with a thirty-year history of hospitalizations and treatment for paranoid schizophrenia, he talked about how his family and guardian were out to get him and had deemed him incompetent. He abruptly stopped talking after the therapist posed a question and said, "Well, I think that I have talked about all that I need to, and I won't need to be coming back. All mental health professionals just defend abusers like my guardian." When asked what specifically this therapist had said that made him think she was defending the guardian, he was unable to specify and just repeated about everyone defending his guardian and other abusers.

> *Therapist:* So your experience has been that others tend to defend those who have hurt you and that they don't believe you?
> *Client:* Yes, that's right.
> *Therapist:* I wonder if you have almost come to expect that people will react that way.
> *Client:* Well, (*pause*) yes.
> *Therapist:* And it seems that you are thinking that I am, too, even though it is not my intention to defend your guardian. I just am trying to understand what is going on for you and maybe see if I can assist in some way. But it seems that you are judging me, assuming I am like those others without checking to see if it is true.
> *Client:* (*looks startled*) You mean like jumping to conclusions?
> *Therapist:* Yes. And given your experience, it seems very important that you and I check with each other about what we are thinking and what we mean so that we don't judge one another. What do you think?
> *Client:* Yes, I see what you mean.

In addition to being clear with the client what the therapist was NOT thinking, she also challenged the defense of paranoid projection by returning it to the client and pointing out how he was judging rather than others were judging him. This brought him a step closer to what he was defending against, namely, acknowledging and judging the many problems that he has had that led to needing a guardian.

Another individual who was expressing frustration at his continued stay at the hospital noted that others were trying to put thoughts in his head of poisoning himself.

> *Therapist:* I can see that you are frustrated by still being at the hospital and that is understandable. Sometimes when people get frustrated, they start to think about hurting or killing themselves.
> *Client:* Yeah.
> *Therapist:* I'm wondering if maybe you have ever thought about that.

The client agreed and began to talk about his own frustrations and occasional thoughts to give up.

During a brief, more lucid moment early in therapy, a woman tormented for decades by persecutory auditory hallucinations announced one of her goals for therapy.

> *Client:* I want to help you not be afraid of the voices.
> *Therapist:* I'm not afraid of your voices.
> *Client:* Oh. (*Pause*) Then maybe you should help me.

Therapist:	Are you afraid of the voices?
Client:	Yes.
Therapist:	Then you and I can work on that.

Reversing the projection of anger and potential aggression underlying a client's threats can also be effective. This is done by asking whether the client can be trusted to manage himself to discuss what is going on. This changes the question from whether the client can trust the therapist to whether the therapist can trust the client, thereby returning the projection. In this way, the individual is reassured of his ability to protect himself as well as to manage and express feelings. For example, with an agitated person who loudly expresses that he cannot trust others and may be displaying evidence of potential aggression, the person intervening might say, "What you have to say is important and I am interested in talking with you and understanding what is going on for you. Clearly you are capable of protecting yourself. But can you trust yourself and can I trust you to be able to manage yourself, and to sit safely and discuss this?"

Conclusions

In summary, mental health services for individuals in the Existing Phase begins when the person is functioning well enough to start to examine themselves, their relationships, and their experiences more closely, including thoughts, feelings, and symptoms, with the focus on increasing insight into their difficulties and teaching new strategies for coping. During the Existing Phase, the individual begins to move out of the constant panic of wondering whether s/he exists toward efforts to "get by." The client's sense of threat lessens, but remains. The goal is to increase the individual's capacity to explore a range of activities and expand emotionally, interpersonally, and functionally into the fuller experiences of the Living Phase.

Chapter 4

The Living Phase
Characteristics and care

"I want to have a full and meaningful life."

Characteristics of the person in the Living Phase

The overarching goal of treatment for psychosis is to help individuals move into the Living Phase, where it feels safe to engage more fully with the world, to experience a full range of emotions, to try new activities, to introspect in a deeper way, and to participate in deeper, more meaningful relationships. The Living Phase is characterized by a better differentiated sense of self with significantly less fear of merger, increased accuracy in appraisal of events, and a concomitant lowered arousal level. The individual is able to "think about thinking" and better describe emotional experiences. More reality-based coping, with less retreat into hallucinations or delusions, as well as greater interpersonal awareness and empathy is displayed. In some aspects, the Living Phase is similar to the "adaptive plateau" phase described by Fenton (2000) and the "advanced phase" described in *Personal Therapy* (Hogarty, 2002), where the individual has "the energy for resuming a fuller social and vocational life" and therapy focuses on teaching strategies for "a safe and rewarding reintegration in the community." It is an opportunity for consolidating gains, maintaining progress, and furthering growth.

To be in the Living Phase is to feel safe to more extensively experience the self, relationships with others, and the world. Nonetheless, fears of being overwhelmed by strong affect, of reverting to psychotic responses under stress, and of being harmed by others remain ongoing struggles for individuals with severe psychosis as they progress, rendering it difficult for them to move into the broader, richer experiences affectively, interpersonally, and psychologically of the Living Phase. For example, after years in a psychiatric hospital for chronic, paranoid schizophrenia, a woman gradually grew stronger and more reality-focused, moved into an apartment in the community, and began a community job. Currently, in her work, she is able to provide and express concern for her clients and she has also developed some friendships. She remains careful about her level of stress, however, and does not allow herself to feel things too intensely, for fear of provoking a psychotic regression. Her gradual move from within herself to more interactions and experiences is reflective of the initial stages of the Living Phase. Individuals who experience a first-episode psychosis or less developed forms of psychosis may rebound to the Living Phase more readily, particularly with early intervention, than those who have struggled for extended periods within the Surviving or Existing Phases.

Characteristics of care in the Living Phase

Interventions in this phase build upon the work conducted in the earlier phases and, because individuals in the Living Phase display relatively greater ego strength, interventions may more closely approximate psychotherapy with higher functioning individuals, with increased emphasis on working collaboratively with the therapist, exploring interpersonal issues, more intensive emotional and cognitive work, and greater use of the therapy relationship. The individual may be better able to explore the past, resulting in fluctuations between a past, present, and future focus in therapy. In addition to further strengthening the self-structure and interpersonal relationships, individuals can benefit from further interventions that fortify psychological resources for coping, such as advanced cognitive and behavioral interventions, mindfulness strategies, and problem-solving techniques. Throughout the therapy, however, it is important to maintain particular sensitivity to times when the individual may revert to concerns of the Surviving Phase, requiring resumed emphasis on reinforcing safety and separateness of the self.

An important caveat for this chapter is that the preponderance of clinical and empirical attention to the psychological treatment of schizophrenia has been on individuals in the Existing Phase. Reported recovery rates for those diagnosed with schizophrenia in Western countries have ranged from nearly half when described as a "favorable outcome" (Harrison *et al.*, 2001) to "rare" when evaluated as "full recovery" (Lauronen *et al.*, 2005), suggesting that fewer individuals diagnosed with schizophrenia and treated using former models of care have reached the Living Phase. However, data indicating more promising outcomes for those with a first-episode psychosis and for those with psychosis treated from a recovery model have catalyzed changes in expectations about prognosis and in treatment approach. The Living Phase is the phase in which we aspire for all people to function, and represents a challenging, but important, goal of treatment for individuals with severe psychosis. The mental health professional must believe that this is possible to be an effective contributor to the progress of the client with psychosis, especially those with severe forms of psychosis. The remainder of this chapter will describe specific elements of psychological interventions for facilitating progress in the Living Phase and to provide guideposts toward which to move in treatment during earlier phases.

Treatment strategies for the Living Phase

Develop a more positive, balanced self-view

As part of continuing to foster self-development, it becomes important to integrate the problems of experiencing severe psychosis into the self-view as one aspect of the person, rather than something that is denied or that becomes the sole basis of identity. Some clinicians have described this as facilitating the individual's acknowledgment of and adjustment to the vulnerabilities and limitations of having schizophrenia, similar to the focus on adjustment to having a disability (Hogarty, 2002). Acknowledgment of the problems associated with severe psychosis is an essential part of relapse prevention, including appropriate self-care and self-monitoring as well as engagement in necessary health behaviors for maintaining progress. However, there is a need to avoid descriptions that suggest the problem is the person's identity (e.g., "I am a schizophrenic") and, instead, facilitate recognition of problems and vulnerabilities that can be addressed (e.g., "I have experienced severe psychosis, at times"). This approach is consistent with contemporary models that discuss psychosis in a way that recognizes various causes and manifestations, instills hope, and engages individuals in actively participating in their treatment planning and recovery.

In addition, in order to promote a more positive self-view, acknowledgment of difficulties needs to be counterbalanced by a focus on the individual's strengths and interests. In particular, continuing to identify interests and encourage activities is an important part of broadening the self-view as an individual with different roles, interests, and strengths rather than being "just a schizophrenic" or a "mental patient." That is, to facilitate the move from "patienthood to personhood" (Roe, 2001) requires continuing to expand and fortify the self-structure, with increasing awareness of a complex self. Certainly, the longer a person has been involved in mental health treatment, the more difficult it is to move beyond seeing the self as "sick" or a "mentally ill patient" to a capable, functioning individual who belongs in and contributes to society. In an initial session, one individual expressed wanting to be able to laugh with his therapist, noting, "I want my therapist to see me as a person." His desire to share humor was a poignant example of the yearning for "normal," positive interpersonal relating, and to be experienced as a human being rather than as a diagnosis.

One client simply and succinctly stated that the main problem for individuals as they leave a psychiatric hospital is "confidence," specifically a lack of confidence. Despite being a highly intelligent, musical, talented individual, he had lost belief in his capabilities to do anything that he did prior to hospitalization and was rigidly convinced of a bleak future. An extensive hospitalization (many years) during his early twenties had resulted in an adult identity as someone dependent, helpless, and sick, who wouldn't be capable of functioning or of being safe outside the hospital. With extensive support, he was able to make gradual transitions to therapeutic employment and an apartment on the hospital grounds. Eventually, he was able to transition to an apartment in the community and the hospital's assertive community treatment program while continuing to work on campus. Each step, however small and gradual, he experienced with severe anxiety that often resulted in intensified psychotic experiences of paranoia. His attachment with the hospital (including with his therapist) was one of hostile dependence and recapitulated his experience with his mother. Similar to his childhood relationship with his mother, he believed he needed the hospital in order to survive, which necessitated remaining "sick" and incapable. Getting stronger and healthier would mean abandonment. This resulted in resentment in his relationship with caregivers and with the institution and appeared to contribute to perpetuation of his psychosis and hospitalization. For him to move into the Living Phase, which he has ventured into but not yet remained in, requires a restructuring of his self-view as well as the nature of his attachments. Part of this does involve building his "confidence" in his abilities and his roles without getting overwhelmed and reverting into psychosis. It also involves developing relationships that don't require he be "ill" or helpless in order to maintain attachments.

This man's slow progress and vulnerability to regression are common in those who have experienced chronic, severe forms of psychosis. For them, regaining a life where psychosis is less interfering and life is more fulfilling is possible, but likely will be accompanied by residual psychological scars and vulnerabilities. These "scars" either can be viewed as imperfections or regarded as symbols of what the person has had the strength to survive. Acknowledgment and integration of traumatic events, including distressing psychosis, as well as related, residual vulnerabilities, into the broader definition of a person and his/her life experience is an important part of remaining in the Living Phase.

Other individuals are able to expand their self-view more readily than the prior example, particularly if they have experienced briefer or less severe forms of psychosis. A broader self-view can be accelerated as individuals increase their interactions in community settings, such as through work environments, churches, and social organizations, and discover that they can relate to people (and obtain support) based on interests rather than on psychiatric problems. Community-based programs facilitate these links to ease the individual back into society. The additional challenges incurred when reintegrating into the community following extended hospitalizations accentuate the need for limiting hospital stays and greater emphasis on community-based treatment whenever possible. Community-based care reduces risks of becoming entrenched in a self-view as a patient and assists the individual in maintaining supports, interests, and other roles.

Continue to provide psychodynamically informed interventions

Research suggests that psychodynamic psychotherapies can be effective for treating psychosis (for a review, see Summers and Rosenbaum, in press). As highlighted throughout this book, psychodynamic approaches are useful in conceptualizing and informing interventions across phases of psychosis. Individuals in the Living Phase, with their improved introspective capacity and ability to better tolerate and manage anxiety, may be more responsive to more exploratory ("uncovering") psychodynamic techniques, such as increasing use of the therapy relationship, encouraging a greater range of emotional expression, and increasing awareness of the effects of past experiences on the individual in the present. This work can be started with individuals later in the Existing Phase as they progress toward the Living Phase. The therapy in the Living Phase, then, can further assist the individual in connecting defenses/responses to the past, expressing related affect, and in coping without regressing into psychotic distortions. Transference reactions that arise and the clinician's counter-transference responses more often can be directly discussed in the therapy, collaboratively exploring the reactions as reflecting the client's self-view as well as her typical expectations and actions within relationships, based on past experiences.

The focus in a session may shift between current relationships with others in the person's life, past relationships, and the current therapeutic relationship, closely monitoring the client's reactions and anxiety level. A frequent occurrence can be a notable change in the amount of engagement the client displays at different times. When a client who has been more actively involved in therapy enters the session more guarded, the therapist may comment: "You seem more distant today, like there is more of a wall between us. Do you notice that?" If there is agreement and the person appears capable of managing some processing of emotional material, joint exploration can occur for possible reasons for the change in trust. For example, "Last time we talked some about how your mother mistreated you when you were a child. I know that she really hurt you and it is understandable that you are more cautious around her. But it seems like it has affected your trust in me, too. It is as if you are expecting that I, also, will hurt you as she did." This validates the person's experience as well as increases the person's awareness of his/her immediate presentation and interaction within the therapy relationship and of a proclivity to generalize mistrust to other relationships. Exploring whether there are specific ways in which the therapist has hurt or not hurt the client might ensue.

Caution must continue to be used in moderating the extent of focus on the immediate relationship according to the person's ability to tolerate the intimacy and emotional intensity. Similarly, interpretations should be used judiciously, as the more fragile individual, even in the Living Phase, may experience an interpretation as too intrusive or commanding. As previously noted, individuals who are experiencing psychosis for the first time or have a less developed form of psychosis may more readily respond to more in-depth explorations than those who are emerging from a severe, longer-term psychosis. Many psychodynamically oriented approaches to psychosis have been described, both in the past (e.g., Fromm-Reichman, 1952; Benedetti, 1980) as well as more recently (e.g., Brent, 2009; Lotterman, 1996).

Continue advanced trauma work

One aspect to exploration of the past, conducted as part of psychodynamic as well as many other theoretical approaches, pertains to exploration of past traumatic experiences. Advanced trauma work often becomes an important part of the therapy in the Living Phase, as research indicates that individuals with psychotic disorders are at least as likely, if not more, to have a history of childhood abuse compared to those with other psychiatric diagnoses (Read *et al.*, 2004). Such work may include emotional processing of traumatic experiences and directly expressing affect related to memories of past painful events. Further, the individual in the Living Phase may be more able to examine psychotic responses as an understandable response (i.e., defense) to actual threats, and work on better distinguishing between actual and perceived threats.

Carefully paced interventions to provide identification and validation of the individual's specific trauma responses, with opportunities for cognitive and emotional processing, may be useful. For example, a modified approach to treating PTSD for those with severe mental illness has shown promise (Ford *et al.*, 2005). Specific trauma effects and personal trauma reminders/triggers can be identified and addressed. In addition, fears of "getting sick again" can continue to contribute to avoidance and restriction of experience, thereby limiting growth and progress. This may be related to psychosocial stressors that prompted past psychotic episodes or to the traumatic experience of the psychotic episode and hospitalization, as manifested in a post-psychotic PTSD (Frame and Morrison, 2001). Details regarding the incorporation of trauma treatment into the therapy are described in Chapter 5.

Further assess for possible dissociative experiences

Part of trauma work in the Living Phase includes continued efforts to help the person identify the ways in which s/he reacts to perceived threats (both internal and external) by distancing or disengaging from the present moment. This is a generalized definition of avoidance strategies that fall under descriptions of psychosis and dissociation and include derealization, emotional numbing, depersonalization, and altered body experiences. It may be easier to begin to identify these types of experiences during the Living Phase because there is reduced interference from hallucinations and delusions, increased logical thinking, and improved self-definition. There also can be greater trust developed within the therapeutic relationship to do the introspective and reflective work necessary. For example, a therapist observed that her client appeared to "go away" briefly in a session when talking about something anxiety-producing for her. The woman was unsure what had happened when asked, but acknowledged that she had not heard what the therapist had been saying. The client and therapist were able to determine how long she had been "disconnected" from the discussion based on what she last recalled in the conversation. She was able to describe other times when a similar experience had occurred and she had "lost time," sometimes extensively and in the absence of psychotic symptoms, such as hearing voices or increased paranoia. The therapist explained the concept of dissociation and noted that, for some people, they start to dissociate as a means of escaping from an otherwise inescapable and frightening experience. To this, the client noted that she thought maybe she had started dissociating as a young girl when her father would tie her down and molest her. She did not elaborate at the time. The therapist did add that, while dissociating sometimes is helpful initially, over time dissociating can become an automatic response to stress that doesn't protect someone as well as staying present. The woman agreed that she wanted to continue to work on ways to stay present instead of dissociating. Issues related to dissociation and psychosis are explored further in Chapter 5. In addition, other sources provide detailed discussions of the relationship between trauma, dissociation, and psychosis (e.g., Moskowitz *et al.*, 2008; Moskowitz, 2011).

Conduct deeper self–other work

As the individual develops more security in the self as a separate person, receptiveness to exploring and engaging in interpersonal relationships may increase. Therapy can increasingly focus on interpersonal experiences, both inside and outside of the therapeutic relationship, to improve social skills and social functioning. Some basic concerns, such as managing the stigma of experiencing psychosis and fielding questions about prior hospitalizations during community interactions, frequently arise as an issue to problem-solve. Deeper issues addressed in therapy pertain to the desire for, but intense vulnerability in, closer relationships that may persist for the individual. Exploration of expectations in relationships, and possible sources of those expectations, facilitates awareness. Additionally, the corrective experience of the therapy relationship and with other treatment professionals begins to modify the person's internal template of self–other relations, and becomes particularly meaningful when these differences are directly discussed. Exploration may include the individual's expectations of others, from where those expectations derive, and what exceptions she/he has experienced in relationships. The caution in relationships can begin to be verbalized more, such as the new client who told her therapist, "I like you so far."

A woman sought outpatient psychotherapy during a marital separation and divorce. At times in the initial phase of therapy, she would describe needing more medication because of increasing paranoia. This was progress in that it demonstrated her awareness of her warning signs and willingness to seek assistance; however, she had difficulty in identifying factors that may have contributed to the increased mistrust, particularly interactions with her former spouse. As therapy progressed and her insight increased, she once started a therapy session by announcing that she had realized that her ex-husband gave her a stomach ache. This was an important realization about the effect that her former spouse had on her, and it made developmental sense that her initial awareness would be of the physical experience of the stress. Later in the same session she asked rather abruptly about side-effects of the antipsychotic she was taking. When queried what her concern was, she initially avoided the question. Eventually she expressed having experienced a reduction in appetite in the past two days, which she thought may be an effect of medication.

> *Therapist:*   And when was the last time you spoke to your ex-husband?
> *Client:*   (*Pausing and then smiling*) About two days ago.
> *Therapist:*   I think that what you may be experiencing is actually side-effects of talking with your ex-husband. Perhaps it might help to problem-solve ways to reduce your dosage of him!
> *Client:*   (*Laughing*) That's very funny.

This discussion reflects the woman's emerging connections between her emotions, her physical reactions, and her relationships. Although she initially identified the physical effect her ex-husband was having on her, she later attributed some of her reactions to medication. The therapist's gentle joking presented the connections in a more palatable and familiar way to the client. She was beginning to move from "I'm sick, I need more medication" to exploring what was upsetting her and finding a variety of ways to address the contributing factors. At times, this might mean modifying her medication regimen, but it also meant a more multi-faceted perspective on her experiences and possible solutions.

Continue family work

The above anecdote also provides an example of the frequent opportunities that arise in therapy in the Living Phase to address family issues. In addition to addressing past difficulties, current goals frequently pertain to how the individual wants to develop more satisfying interactions and communication with family, and learn ways to assert and set limits. Asking "How old do you feel when you are with your parents?" can prompt the realization of regression when with the family of origin and foster discussion of ways to interact with them that feels more consistent with the individual's current age. As discussed previously, if the client lives with family, it is generally indicated to have some family sessions. Family therapy can involve structured problem-solving as well as more emotional processing as the client feels safe enough to do so. However, if the person lives apart from family, even if there is frequent contact, addressing family issues without having the members participate directly in the therapy may serve to continue to bolster the separateness and independence of the client.

Conduct advanced work regarding thought processes

The Living Phase is propitious for cognitive-behavior therapy, given the increased ability to "think about thinking" and greater insight and engagement. As noted by Beck *et al.* (2009: 194), individuals who "have a greater awareness of their thoughts and can readily understand the associations between thoughts, feelings, and behaviors may be more likely to embrace and work within the cognitive model." Interventions in the Surviving and Existing Phases, as described in the previous chapters, can do the necessary foundation work, including increasing awareness of thoughts, introducing connections as well as differences between thoughts, feelings, and actions, and enhancing cognitive flexibility. Those advancing in the Existing Phase toward more characteristics of the Living Phase may begin to do more advanced CBT work that is continued in the Living Phase. Based on readiness in the Living Phase, cognitive restructuring exercises can be conducted as well, both for daily concerns as well as for delusions and hallucinations. Further opportunities in sessions can be created for the individual to learn how to differentiate between facts and perceptions of experiences. Beliefs about the power and validity of voices or about other delusional beliefs can continue to be collaboratively explored and tested with the client. Further honing cognitive appraisals of events will help to reduce the perception of threat, such as addressing reasoning biases and negative schemas that may contribute to the formation and maintenance of delusional beliefs, hallucinations, and interpersonal mistrust (Kuipers *et al.*, 2006). This includes further exploring appraisals of psychotic experiences, particularly hallucinations. For example, an individual in the Living Phase, when he experiences auditory hallucinations, now tells himself, "Oh, I am starting to hear voices again; I must be more stressed about something." He provides himself with a manageable explanation for the experience that does not result in escalating distress and implies that he can do something to help himself. The appraisal returns perceived influence and efficacy to him. In addition, despite progress, research indicating persistent cognitive deficits in persons diagnosed with schizophrenia (O'Carroll, 2000) suggests that many individuals who have progressed to the Living Phase still continue to struggle with deficits in such areas as social cognition, executive functioning, sustained attention, and social competence. Therefore, continued efforts for cognitive remediation remain important for improving functional outcome.

Often, cognitive interventions can remain very simple. For example, one client presented feeling more distressed and paranoid within the context of multiple stressors. In therapy, she and her therapist organized her primary concerns into specific, discrete problems. She then decided that, when she got home, she would write down each problem or issue as well as potential solutions on separate file cards. In this way, she quickly moved from feeling overwhelmed by myriad concerns to developing an active, effective problem-solving approach. It was important for her to determine what the approach would be and to do it privately rather than in session.

Continue to promote reality-based coping

In this phase, individuals may particularly benefit from learning additional skills, including advanced social skills training, mindfulness strategies, and problem-solving techniques. Exploring concerns and experiences that arise as the person increasingly interacts in the community can provide opportunities in therapy for normalizing, psycho-education, in vivo practice (e.g., role-plays), increasing accuracy of appraisal of situations, and bolstering self-confidence. Honing recognition of and adaptive response to personal warning signs of stress and anger remains a critical part of preventing relapse into psychosis. However, increasing awareness of the individual's emotional experience can continue to be difficult, given the tendency to rely on avoidance, denial, and projection. In the Living Phase, the therapeutic relationship can provide more opportunities to safely acknowledge and explore different emotions and learn adaptive means for expressing them. As an example, one individual was in a state psychiatric hospital in the United States for approximately twenty years on a "not guilty by reason of mental illness" status. When he obtained a conditional release to move into the community, he began to experience an increase in anxiety and problems in thinking. He described "episodes" or "events" during which he would feel overcome and would have trouble with his thoughts (unspecified). He noted that he would curl up on his bed and wait for it (the episode) to be over. He could not identify any physical sensations that accompanied these experiences. He was uncomfortable with calling it anxiety or panic attacks, but was receptive to discussing some of the changes occurring in his life and expectable reactions to these changes.

He subsequently was able to explore some of his worries and his thoughts and, later, to problem-solve ways to manage the stress. He later told his case manager that, with the therapist, "I tell her my bizarre thoughts and she helps me make sense of them." Normalizing his increased anxiety and problems in thinking as part of change and progress, identifying "unacceptable" thoughts and feelings that arose during the stress, and developing adaptive ways to cope helped him to continue in the Living Phase.

Group psychotherapies that teach such topics as social skills, stress management, vocational skills, and self-care can augment coping and life skills and complement the work of individual therapy. In addition, for those with co-occurring addictions, advanced substance abuse treatment is an important aspect to relapse prevention as well. More details regarding group therapies are presented in Chapter 6.

Continue to monitor and adjust the psychological space in the therapy relationship as needed

Consistent with work in the Existing Phase, interventions in the Living Phase need to be conducted with particular sensitivity to times when the individual may revert to concerns of the Surviving Phase, requiring resumed emphasis on reinforcing safety and separateness of the self. The therapist must remain alert to client fluctuations in status and promptly and adroitly respond. While the client is in the Existing Phase, the therapist may respond by quickly shifting to less emotionally provoking topics, directly reiterating regarding safety, or emphasizing differentiation to fortify the basic self-structure. In the Living Phase, more efforts are made to increase client awareness of the occurrence of these regressions in the moment or by processing once the client has reconstituted. For example, the therapist may note, "This seems to be a difficult topic to discuss. Do you think we should change the subject for awhile or just breathe for a minute?" In this way, the therapist is able to increase awareness of the effect of a topic in the moment and facilitate reality-based, adaptive coping.

Conclusions

This chapter has described some of the main tenets of psychological interventions for the Living Phase. To date, there has been more clinical and empirical focus on individuals whose psychosis was acute or partially remitted (i.e., in the Surviving or Existing Phase) than on those in the Living Phase. An optimistic perspective on the fewer numbers in the Living Phase would be that individuals in the Living Phase are functioning well enough to not need (or desire) treatment. However, as discussed earlier in the chapter, a more likely explanation is that individuals diagnosed with schizophrenia in Western countries and treated solely with medication have low rates of recovery, resulting in fewer individuals experiencing a severe psychosis progressing to the Living Phase. It may also be that fewer individuals diagnosed with schizophrenia come to therapy when in the Living Phase because, given the ongoing issues with trust and self-other struggles, treatment is not sought unless the level of distress or concern exceeds the level of social discomfort. Fears of being rehospitalized, overmedicated, or misunderstood may also serve as barriers to psychotherapy and to mental health care in general. Additionally, even the Existing Phase can seem good in comparison to the experiences of complete regression into the Surviving Phase, much like purgatory would be experienced as an improvement if one had been living in hell. The hope is that, with active, phase-specific, recovery-oriented care, more individuals with psychosis will progress to a point where they are more fully living, rather than merely surviving or existing.

Chapter 5

Incorporating trauma treatment into care for psychosis

"I've been invaded my whole life."

There is increasing recognition that traumatic experiences and trauma responses are a significant part of severe psychosis, and this awareness is contributing to a shift in conceptualization of and approach to the psychoses. The extensive advances in trauma treatment can be adapted to trauma-informed treatment for severe psychosis, including schizophrenia (Fuller, 2010). To this end, this chapter will describe the incorporation of trauma treatment principles into psychological interventions for psychosis across the Surviving, Existing, and Living Phases. In order to provide a foundation on which to discuss this, first the relationship between trauma and psychosis and aspects of general trauma treatment are discussed.

The relationship between trauma and psychosis

It is often easy to see the individual with severe psychosis as traumatized, by the psychotic experience itself and, often, by past events the psychosis may defend against or represent. Individuals diagnosed with schizophrenia have high rates of abuse histories and many display difficulties that are consistent with trauma responses described in the literature, including greater reactivity to stress, hypervigilance, interpersonal distrust, cognitive difficulties, intrusive thoughts and memories, emotional restriction, dissociation, and a feeling of detachment. In addition, hallucinations often have elements of actual traumatic experiences, such as hearing the voice of an abuser. Paranoia can have its roots in actual harm by others. When the therapist looks beyond a diagnosis of schizophrenia, often the individual can be understood as presenting with extreme trauma responses. Indeed, PTSD is frequently co-morbid with schizophrenia, with the rate of current PTSD for those with a diagnosis of schizophrenia being approximately 27 to 29 percent (Resnick *et al.*, 2003; Sarkar *et al.*, 2005). This rate far exceeds the current rate of 3.5 percent for the general population (Kessler *et al.*, 2005).

Psychotic symptoms clearly can develop in response to life-threatening events and other traumatic experiences. For example, approximately one-third of Vietnam veterans diagnosed with Posttraumatic Stress Disorder (PTSD) experience some hallucinations and/or delusions (Seedat *et al.*, 2003). Inclusion of the diagnosis of Brief Psychotic Disorder with Marked Stressor in the DSM-IV-TR (American Psychiatric Association, 2000) also supports the causal role of traumatic events in the development of psychosis. Other evidence for the role of traumatic experiences in the development of psychosis comes from prospective and population-based studies, which have found childhood interpersonal traumas to be a significant predictor of psychosis, even after controlling for many potentially confounding factors, including family history of psychosis. For example, results of one large-scale study indicated that subjects who had a history of childhood physical or sexual abuse were more than nine times more likely to have developed psychotic symptoms over time compared to those without an abuse history, even after controlling for psychiatric diagnosis, education, economic status, age, gender, substance abuse history, and history of positive psychotic symptoms or mental health treatment in first-degree relatives (Janssen *et al.*, 2004). As another example, a longitudinal, prospective twin study found that children's report of psychotic symptoms was strongly associated with childhood interpersonal trauma, both bullying by peers and abuse perpetrated by adults, controlling for genetic proneness to psychosis (Arseneault *et al.*, 2011).

Such data indicate that traumatic events can play a role in the development of psychosis. The reverse is also true. That is, a psychotic episode can be a traumatizing experience and result in trauma responses. Specifically, research indicates that many individuals develop PTSD symptoms in response to the trauma of a psychotic episode and/or of hospitalization, with rates of what is being referred to as Postpsychotic PTSD (PP/PTSD) as high as 52 percent (Frame and Morrison, 2001; McGorry *et al.*, 1991; Shaw *et al.*, 2002). This is not surprising when an acute psychotic episode in severe psychosis is recognized as an intense threat to self-integrity and to existence. Furthermore, a psychotic episode can challenge the person's beliefs about themselves, others, and the world (Davidson and Strauss, 1992). Hospitalization for a psychotic episode may also add to stress responses by furthering the sense of victimization, threat, and helplessness (Beveridge, 1998). Finally, the consequent extensive efforts to avoid affective, cognitive, and situational reminders of the psychotic episode (Shaner and Eth, 1989) also are consistent with PTSD.

Yet, despite high rates of abuse in those diagnosed with schizophrenia, the overlap in trauma responses and psychotic symptoms, and the rates of PTSD in those diagnosed with schizophrenia, schizophrenia continues to be primarily discussed and treated as an inherited brain disorder, with PTSD symptoms and other stress-related responses either disregarded, minimized, or viewed only as sequelae of schizophrenia. In contrast, although individuals with Dissociative Identity Disorder (DID) report more first-rank symptoms of schizophrenia than people diagnosed with schizophrenia (Kluft, 1987; Ross *et al.*, 1990), DID is conceptualized as an environmentally caused disorder that develops in response to adverse life events. These vastly different perspectives or "opposing paradigms" (Moskowitz, 2011) result in very different treatment approaches, with schizophrenia primarily treated pharmacologically and DID with psychological interventions.

A return to the stress-vulnerability model (Zubin and Spring, 1977) dissolves this dichotomy and yields a more comprehensive understanding of the relationship between trauma and psychosis. Generally, application of this model to psychosis has been interpreted to mean that genetic predispositions may be triggered by sufficient psychosocial/environmental stressors, which then result in psychosis. However, Zubin and Spring (1977) also proposed that vulnerability to psychosis could be *acquired* in response to such events as trauma, family experiences, and perinatal factors, not just inherited. In support, the flourishing research into the neurobiology of trauma has yielded strong evidence that biological vulnerability for psychosis can be acquired in response to adverse life experiences. Read *et al.* (2008) postulated that prolonged exposure to adverse childhood events results in an alteration in the brain's stress regulation mechanisms, thereby creating the neurological and biochemical differences often cited as evidence of schizophrenia being a brain disease. Alterations in the hypothalamic-pituitary-adrenal axis due to trauma may result in one mechanism by which vulnerability to psychosis is acquired (Cotter and Pariente, 2002). Accumulating data also indicate that childhood abuse adversely affects the developing brain by lowering the threshold for neurobiological stress responses (Vasterling and Brewin, 2005). Furthermore, structural deviations – such as enlarged ventricles and reduced cerebral size – which are often cited as evidence of structural differences in the brains of persons diagnosed with schizophrenia, have also been described in children who have been traumatized (DeBellis *et al.*, 2005) and in adults with PTSD (Gilbertson *et al.*, 2002). Such neurobiological research provides evidence that vulnerability to develop psychosis can be acquired through life experience and indicates that psychosocial factors may contribute on both "sides" of the stress-vulnerability model, as either a predisposing or an activating factor. This perspective necessitates implicit acceptance of a biopsychosocial approach to understanding severe psychosis, including schizophrenia.

In summary, there is a strong body of evidence indicating a relationship between trauma and psychosis, with accumulating empirical support for the role of trauma as a cause and/or consequence of psychosis. Comprehensive approaches to trauma-related disorders recognize the environmental factors that contribute to the development of stress responses and attend to psychological, physiological, interpersonal, self, and spiritual effects of the trauma in treatment. Yet, despite the documented high rates of childhood abuse in individuals diagnosed with schizophrenia, mental health professionals are less likely to assess for a history of childhood abuse in individuals diagnosed with schizophrenia than with other disorders (Read and Fraser, 1998). In addition, individuals diagnosed with schizophrenia often do not receive a co-morbid diagnosis of PTSD, despite meeting criteria (Mueser *et al.*, 1998). This may be partially attributable to the difficulty in differentiating trauma responses from positive and negative symptoms of psychosis, but also stems from continued perseverance of a purely biological perspective of schizophrenia.

Complete treatment for severe psychosis needs to incorporate trauma-sensitive and trauma-targeted interventions. This is particularly important given that traumatic events can be associated with greater chronicity and severity of psychotic symptoms, as well as with greater functional impairment (Lysaker *et al.*, 2001; Mueser *et al.*, 2004). However, the limited empirical and clinical attention and training related to trauma treatment for this population has left therapists with inadequate guidance on an effective approach. Other barriers to trauma assessment and intervention have included fear of exacerbating client distress by asking about a potentially emotionally provoking topic or having other treatment priorities, such as stabilization during brief hospitalization (Young *et al.*, 2001). Particularly in outpatient settings, therapists are often reluctant to address trauma-related issues for fear of destabilizing the individual. The largest barrier to trauma-informed treatment, however, has been the prior, stalwart genetic position for schizophrenia. Recognition of the role of traumatic life experiences in severe psychosis necessitates a dramatic alteration in our understanding of etiology as well as treatment. Fortunately, this advance in perspective humanizes what is often a dehumanizing condition.

Primary elements of trauma treatment

Advances in general trauma treatment lay the groundwork for developing effective trauma-based interventions for severe psychosis. The typical, initial objectives of trauma treatment with an acutely distressed individual are pertinent for those experiencing acute psychosis as well: increase the sense of safety, attend to basic needs, stabilize and support the person, bolster coping, and reduce distress (National Child Traumatic Stress Network and National Center for PTSD, 2007). In addition, one of the first steps in trauma treatment is the determination of whether or not the threat (i.e., the event prompting the trauma responses) is over (Briere and Scott, 2006). If it is not over, the therapist provides support and assists in developing ways to increase the sense of safety, such as through the development of a safety plan. For example, a safety plan for a woman currently in a domestically violent relationship might include always having a cell phone in her possession, having the number of a safe house, and keeping essentials (such as medications and money) in an accessible, alternative location to her home. If an actual threat no longer exists, the therapist assists the individual in improving threat perception and distinguishing past from present concerns. Once perceived or actual threat is reduced, psycho-education about PTSD and enhancing coping skills can assist in stabilizing and strengthening the individual to manage both immediate stressors as well as stressors related to past traumatic events. Finally, after the individual perceives a greater sense of safety and is more stable, methods for processing traumatic memories can be conducted.

For trauma treatment in general as well as specifically for severe psychosis, delivering trauma-specific interventions based on the individual's psychological readiness is essential for maximizing effectiveness as well as for minimizing risk of destabilization. Although specific interventions vary, many trauma treatment models first focus on safety and stabilization, followed by psycho-education and skill building, before processing and integration work. These general phases in trauma treatment can be integrated into psychological treatment over the course of severe psychosis based on whether the individual is in the Surviving, Existing, or Living Phase. Generally, the

Surviving Phase targets reduction of acute distress (stabilization) and increasing the sense of safety. Introductory trauma work, including education regarding trauma effects and enhancing coping skills, can be conducted for those in the Existing Phase, with more advanced trauma work (e.g., exploration and processing of traumatic events, additional skill building) implemented in the Living Phase. The remainder of the chapter provides details of applications of trauma treatment during the different phases of severe psychosis.

Trauma-related interventions during the Surviving Phase

During the Surviving Phase of severe psychosis, the focus of treatment shares the goals of initial trauma treatment of promoting safety and stability. In addition to providing support, bolstering coping, and assisting with basic needs, specific places, activities, and people may be designated as helpful for increasing a sense of protection. For those persons in the community, a safety plan also may involve knowing that hospitalization is available, if needed. However, this is reassuring for some individuals, but terrifying for others. Inpatient safety plans may involve identifying specific places and people within the hospital that feel more secure.

As with any acutely distressed, traumatized individual, frequently the psychological and physiological reactions to stimuli can be as if a past threat is a current one. Hypervigilance and hypersensitivity to stress reflect that the body and mind continue to be on "high alert." Therefore, as noted earlier in the chapter, the first objective is to ascertain whether the threat is over. With the acutely psychotic individual, however, it can be difficult to clearly determine the extent to which currently perceived threats are accurately appraised or represent a distortion of a past event. The importance of attending to a person's expressed fears is underscored by the fact that the self-report of traumatic events in individuals with severe mental illness has been found to be reliable over time and corroborated by collateral information (Goodman et al., 1999; Read et al., 2003). In addition to direct report, individuals may indirectly communicate about traumatic experiences through delusional material, interpersonal mistrust, and through the content of hallucinations. Consistent with earlier psychodynamic conceptualizations, current cognitive therapy emphasizes that delusions and hallucinations have meaning for the individual and often are related to pre-morbid experiences (e.g., Kingdon and Turkington, 1994). Content of hallucinations and delusions has frequently been found to be related to past trauma, such as childhood abuse (Beck and Van der Kolk, 1987; Calvert et al., 2008). For example, voices that constantly berated one client eventually were understood to recreate bullying experiences he had as a child. Fears of being choked or being penetrated in some way or having bodily organs invaded also can reflect actual experiences of abuse. Auditory hallucinations can be understood as severe trauma responses reflecting intrusive memories, an ongoing sense of threat of harm, or projected feelings of anger, hurt, shame, or fear. Hallucinations and delusions also can replay traumatic events much like flashbacks, resulting in a loss of boundaries between past and present.

Given that the majority of individuals diagnosed with schizophrenia have had traumatic experiences, reassurance of safety often involves acknowledgment and validation of actual threats from the past as well as highlighting increased safety in the present. Further, recognition and commendation that the person managed to survive whatever the difficult event involved highlights his/her capabilities. In addition, emphasis is placed on the fact that the traumatic event occurred in the past, is over, and does not constitute a current threat. This clear distinction between past and present is important for promoting a sense of safety and starting to reduce the ongoing, automatic physiological response of sustained high alert. For example, one woman responded to a persecutory auditory hallucination which she referred to by her father's name. It was easy to conceptualize this voice as reflecting her memories/perception of how her father had talked to her and treated her. When she appeared distressed and would make comments such as "I have to take my punishments," the therapist would respond, "The time of taking punishments is over. You got through that time, you did what you had to in order to get through it, and you are a very brave person. Your father lives far away and he is not allowed to visit. You are safe and protected now." The first time the therapist made such comments, the woman stopped arguing with her voices, looked at the therapist, and smiled broadly.

Such interventions affirm past experiences, but separate them from the present, fortify the individual, and reassure of safety. In this example, the voices the woman heard perpetuated her experience of being abused. General statements such as, "That happened when you were 6 years old. Now you are an adult and can protect yourself better than you could then," also validate the past, distinguish the past from the present, and bolster the belief in the person's current ability to self-protect. During group and individual sessions, the therapist also can ask clients to identify what immediate threats to physical safety exist in the room, address if there are any concerns expressed, and facilitate reality-based assessment. Often, individuals experience some reduction in anxiety when they are anchored (albeit sometimes only briefly) to the moment with a realization that there are no immediate threats.

Enhancing accuracy of threat perception is an ongoing process. Often, it is helpful to repeatedly identify what the perceived threat is and clarify the extent to which it is an actual threat. For example, one woman returned from a billiards club frightened and saying that men were wanting to rape her. Within rapid speech about being raped, she mentioned men waving pool sticks around and trying to hit her. The therapist highlighted the client's immediate safety in the therapy room, ensured and then reassured that she had not been harmed at the clubhouse, and then elicited specific facts about what the men were doing (playing pool), the number of times she had observed them in the past and not been hurt, and what staff were there that could assure her of her safety. Other actions she could take to feel safer (e.g., have a table between her and her peers) were also discussed. For this woman, who had previously reported being raped when she was younger, observing male peers playing pool had prompted fears of being harmed. Distinctions between past and present and reassurance of safety in session were part of increasing her accuracy in threat perception.

In addition to increasing the sense of safety, strategies described in Chapter 2 can be used to reduce physical and emotional arousal and enhance perceived physical and psychological safety, including orienting and grounding, deep breathing, and mindfulness strategies. Medications that reduce anxiety may also prove beneficial. For some, a weighted blanket can also facilitate a sense of safety and containment. An emphasis on the present is important in therapy for both acute psychosis and acute trauma-related distress. In addition, talking about the future when the person will be doing better instills hope and temporarily moves the person away from the past and present to a more manageable future. For example: "You can get to a point where you don't feel so on edge all the time and on high alert. I can see a time in the future where you can know that you are okay and find things more manageable and less frightening." Also, "You can discover that some people can assist you and care about you without harming you." These projections of the future are phrased in such a way as to describe progress, but not be too discrepant from the individual's current status so that the objectives can seem plausible. If the future vision is too discordant with the individual's current perspective, s/he will be more likely to discount it. These positive, future-focused statements convey the therapist's belief in the person's ability to get better, allude to the temporary nature of the problems, and introduce positive expectancy.

Another challenge to trauma-focused treatment for this population is that it is common for a psychotic individual to appear distracted, but sometimes it is difficult to ascertain if it is due to a focus of attention on internal stimuli (e.g., listening to auditory hallucinations) or some other alteration in consciousness. A growing body of research highlights the significant overlap between dissociative symptoms and the positive symptoms of schizophrenia, particularly derealization, depersonalization, and emotional numbing (Ellason and Ross, 1995; Schafer *et al.*, 2008), and indicates that dissociation is a defense frequently displayed by psychotic individuals. This is exemplified in the frequent experience of the psychotic individual of feeling disconnected from his or her body, of cognitive lapses and not remembering, and of the more extreme experience of feeling without a soul. A man described the occasional experience of a famous actor taking over his body and "looking out through my face," reflecting derealization as well as intrusion and permeability. Also similar to dissociation, hallucinations and delusions can be viewed as avoidance strategies, an escape from what is perceived to be intolerable or a breaking off of an unacceptable impulse, feeling, or memory, or a re-experiencing of a traumatic situation. In addition, hallucinations and delusions, like dissociative reactions, can become automatic, unconscious responses over time, providing a brief retreat from perceived internal or external threats. One male client, as he progressed in therapy, noted, "I don't like reality. It is too much for me. People take advantage of me in reality. I choose to stay disconnected from reality." These statements underscore the purpose of and similarities between dissociation and psychosis.

Despite the significant overlap in symptom presentation and trauma histories, clinical perspectives have tended to assume dissociation is trauma-based, but psychosis is of a genetic origin. Fortunately, the shared symptoms are responsive to interventions focused on reorienting the client, increasing the sense of safety, and differentiating past from present. A shared goal is to assist the client in discovering that remaining present is better protection than the strategy of "going away" either by listening to hallucinatory voices or by other ways of disengaging from the present moment (e.g., depersonalization and derealization). This is first addressed in the Surviving Phase by "grounding" the person in the immediate situation and by using other reality orientation strategies. Grounding techniques involve utilizing all of the senses as well as reassurances to help the person return their focus to the immediate location and situation. "You are just right here in the room with me and you are okay. Can you feel your feet on the floor? Start to move your right foot, now your left foot." Instructing the individual to look around the room, to notice things, and to look at you, concurrent with reassurances about their safety, facilitates a safe return to the moment. Movement also assists in interrupting the physiological "freeze" response.

Trauma-influenced transference, such as fears of being revictimized by the therapist, need to be directly addressed and assuaged. For example, the woman whose auditory hallucination was referred to by her father's name was informed, "When someone is hurt badly by someone else, it is common for them to worry that others will hurt them, too. I want you to know that I will not hurt you the way your father did and I will show you that by my words and by my actions." In another case, a man mentioned in Chapter 3 had described his mother as being inappropriate in her boundaries ("I think she is in love with me"). When the man went on a home visit to his mother's residence, he became very paranoid and distressed and reported that his mother had been making sexual advances. While the veracity of his concerns could not be substantiated, he was in acute psychotic distress related to his experience. When his ongoing therapist met with him upon his return, he expressed in the midst of rapid, often difficult to comprehend, speech that the therapist was sexually interested in him. He was reassured of the boundaries with clear statements such as, "You and I just talk and nothing sexual is going to happen. I express my interest in and concern for you only in words."

Consistent with the general trauma literature, intensive exploration of thoughts, feelings, and memories with the psychotic individual is not conducted during the Surviving Phase. Generally, such processing is discouraged when the person is still in an unsafe situation and/or is highly distressed (Ford et al., 2005; Shalev et al., 2000) as it may exacerbate reactions and further overwhelm coping resources. Postponement of processing until the person is more stable is advisable not only because of the high distress of the Surviving Phase, but also because of the deficits of an acute phase of severe psychosis, including schizophrenia, previously discussed, including alexithymia (a limited ability to cognitively construct and process emotions), limited awareness of thoughts, and an internal focus that limits awareness of and connection with others (Cullberg, 2006). Therefore, more extensive cognitive and emotional trauma work needs to be delayed until the individual displays requisite capacities to explore and address thoughts and feelings.

Trauma-related interventions during the Existing Phase

As discussed in previous chapters, an individual's move into the Existing Phase is characterized by improvements in the person's sense of safety, reality orientation, and engagement in treatment, as well as increased cognitive, emotional and interpersonal awareness, and a more coherent self-perception. As these features of improved functioning re-emerge, additional aspects of trauma treatment can be introduced to further reduce stress-related responses. For example, psycho-education about trauma-related stress responses can augment similar education that normalizes and explains psychotic responses. Specific skills can be taught for lowering arousal, coping with stressors, and improving self-regulation, as described in interventions for schizophrenia as well as for PTSD and other trauma-related disorders (Linehan, 1993; Rothbaum et al., 2000). These skills include emotion identification and labeling of emotions without judging (e.g., "that is just my body responding to stress"), relaxation strategies, mindfulness techniques, cognitive reframing, positive self-coaching, and enhancing basic self-care through exercise and improved nutrition.

Although relaxation strategies are essential, such strategies require introspection as well as a willingness to reduce guardedness and hypervigilance. Specifically, the person has to be willing to reflect upon his internal state and acknowledge his emotional experience: something the person with severe psychosis tends to avoid. In addition, the person has to believe that lowering arousal is indicated and can be more protective than remaining vigilant. The traumatized person often becomes accustomed to hyperarousal and hypervigilance as a means of being on guard and feeling protected. Hypervigilance allows a person to actively watch out for and be ready to respond to anticipated threats. Consequently, suggestions to lower arousal can be perceived as encouragement to be vulnerable. It is like asking the person in a castle who is anticipating the approach of an enemy to remove the sentries from the lookout tower and to open the drawbridge. Being calm and relaxed means believing that one can trust the self, others, and the environment not to be harmful; that the situation is safe. As the person becomes better able to accurately assess what actual threats currently exist and what his reactions are, he will concomitantly be better able to discern when it is appropriate and actually more protective to "lower the drawbridge." A particular challenge for the therapist, then, is to create opportunities to help the client realize that calmly and directly addressing many emotionally charged situations and memories can be more effective and protective than hyper-aroused avoidance.

Another challenge to teaching self-monitoring and relaxation strategies is that physiological and emotional arousal in the traumatized individual, including those with severe psychosis, sometimes is not easy to detect. Often, an individual may look and experience more numbness and disconnection from affect than distress; what is often referred to as the "freeze" response. Additionally, the person may have learned that not showing emotion was safer or that acknowledgment of emotional experience will lead to being overwhelmed. This disconnection from affect often remains true in the Existing Phase, where distress may have lessened, but emotional experience remains restricted. Repeatedly, clients state that they are not stressed or affected by difficult situations, when their circumstances would predict otherwise. They may report being "good" or "fine" or unclear. Individuals may state what they think they "should" feel or revert to delusional beliefs that elevate mood. For example, one member of a PTSD group who was diagnosed with schizophrenia reflected, "When I get really stressed, I go into this kind of delusional wonderland. I think because it is happier than my real life."

Such a statement also highlights that psychosis can be experienced as a safe retreat from the threats of the real world. A client with a sexual abuse history and severe psychosis stated, "People want to be invanishable." When the therapist queried what "invanishable" meant the client replied, "To have thicker skin and no one can cut you with a knife." The therapist reassured the client about the importance of being able to protect himself and noted, "You have skin that protects you, you are a tall, strong adult male, and you also have staff here to help protect you." The neologism "invanishable" can be viewed as a poignant blend of "vanishable" and "invulnerable" (unable to be harmed), both of which a retreat into psychosis might appear to provide. Psychosis allows one to disappear from reality in order to be unharmed or, at least, less harmed.

Certainly, often hallucinations are persecutory in nature and can torment an individual. In those presentations, it is difficult to imagine that the psychotic experience provides an escape. Nonetheless, even if the hallucinations or beliefs are distressing, they may serve to avoid what is perceived to be even more threatening. Such primitive defenses, as described by McWilliams (1994), "protect the psychotic person against a level of abject dread so overwhelming that even the frightening distortions that the defenses themselves often create are a lesser evil." In such cases, psychosis may serve to avoid experiencing what are perceived to be threatening feelings or impulses. Psychosis also may replay past traumatic experiences in an attempt to work through painful memories and may seem less threatening than being subjected to new, potentially unknown threats.

The perceived benefits of hypervigilance, avoidance, and denial can all interfere with engaging a person in the Existing Phase to employ stress reduction strategies. As a result, individuals often are more receptive to medications than to focusing on their physical state and calming themselves. Therefore, repeated information and in-session experience is needed to highlight the benefits of improved awareness of one's emotional and cognitive state and of lowering overall arousal level. A quantitative rating of stress level from 1 to 10, described in detail in Chapter 6, is an excellent introduction to self-monitoring. Even efforts to increase awareness of thoughts and self-talk can be threatening to the individual who has staunchly avoided and denied internal experiences and internal dialogue. Identifying effective attributes of a coach and employing those techniques to coaching one's self can be used as an alternative descriptor of self-talk. Experiencing the benefits of directly discussing and dealing with minor, daily stressors prepares the client for addressing more difficult situations in the same manner. In this way, self-monitoring can become self-protective and reduce the need for avoidance, denial, and projection of affective and cognitive experiences. Regarding calming strategies, activities that emphasize an external focus, such as distraction techniques (e.g., watching the second hand on a clock), exercise, and other stress-reducing activities (e.g., bathing or showering) initially may be more effective than deep breathing, muscle relaxation, or cognitive techniques that require an internal focus. Such educational and activity-based (experiential) interventions will need to be ongoing for the traumatized individual to truly believe that it can be safer and more effective to self-monitor and to be calmer rather than to be "on guard."

In addition, the grounding and orientation techniques described earlier for the Surviving Phase continue to be utilized in the Existing and Living Phases, with efforts to highlight how remaining present is more protective than "going away." In addition to utilizing movement and engaging the senses to be mindful of the present moment, more can be said to the person in the Existing Phase about the benefits of dealing directly with concerns. One individual in residential treatment began to regress and slip into psychosis under the stress of a potential move into the community. He was told by his therapist, "I can see you becoming more withdrawn into yourself and less trusting in response to the stress of moving. It is understandable that you feel some stress about the change. I want to help you remember that you can better deal with and address the problems that are coming up right now by remaining present and directly dealing with them. You have many people here that can help you through this. You don't have to go away and retreat inside yourself like you have in the past. You are able to handle this."

Another critical aspect of trauma-sensitive therapy in the Existing Phase is to begin to explore the development and meaning of hallucinations and delusions as they relate to past traumatic experiences. These interventions advance the work initiated in the Surviving Phase, which was predicated upon acknowledgment that unresolved traumatic issues can be indirectly expressed through psychotic symptoms. Therapy objectives in the Existing Phase include increasing awareness of any historical or affective roots to an individual's hallucinations or delusions, with the goal of gradually moving the perception from an external to an internal source. This is achieved first by normalizing and providing education about common responses to stressors and then exploring whether a hallucination or delusion reflects an actual memory or certain difficult emotions and facilitating the individual's acknowledgment and acceptance. That is, interventions target reintegrating whatever the hallucination or delusion represents from an externalized perceptual disturbance to one that is acknowledged, internalized, and integrated in the person's life experience. This process is consistent with what has been described as interpretation of projections (Alanen, 1997; Beck, 1952) and more recently described as addressing faulty source monitoring (Garety *et al.*, 2001; Henquet *et al.*, 2005).

As an example, for years a man had interjected comments about "the fifth grade" within rapid, difficult-to-follow speech whenever he was more distressed and psychotic. His extensive psychiatric records noted delusional beliefs and perseverations about elementary school for this man, then in his fifties. In therapy, his feelings of being an outcast, expectations of being judged, and fears of caring about others and being cared about were acknowledged and validated. Over the course of therapy in the Existing Phase, he was able to begin to put together the fragments of memories of an incident of being bullied in his childhood. Discussion of the traumatic event was piecemeal and more general, establishing an outline of the experience through flashes of images, feelings, and thoughts that would be filled in with details once in the Living Phase. He was also able to acknowledge that the voices he heard sometimes said negative things about him that he believed. This recognition was essential groundwork for internalizing unwanted memories and affect that had been projected into taunting, derogatory voices.

Another client was terrified that he would say aloud sexually inappropriate things about children that voices in his head were saying. This frightened him to the extent that it significantly limited his activities and interactions and frequently occupied his thoughts. Eventually, he revealed a belief that all those who were sexually abused as children became perpetrators and was dubious when told statistics indicating otherwise. He acknowledged a history of past sexual abuse, but would not elaborate at that time. He did not have a history of molesting children and assessment did not indicate risk for offending. His therapist provided limited information (based on his tolerance) about potential effects of abuse, normalized transient thoughts that everyone has but does not express or act upon, and reiterated the privacy of thoughts. This client's belief and fear partly arose from his permeability, including lacking distinction between his thoughts and his self and between thoughts and actions. However, his avoidance of painful past experiences also resulted in intrusive, re-experiencing thoughts and fears. The goal was to have the client be able to acknowledge that he is afraid that he will harm children in the way that he was harmed.

As highlighted in the previous examples, past experiences may be carefully explored in the Existing Phase, although it remains important to clearly distinguish past events from the present experiences. For example, one hospitalized man came to session highly distressed and indicated that, when eating lunch at the cafeteria that day, he had seen the man who sexually abused him as a child. The client presented in session as childlike. The therapist calculated the number of years since the client had actually seen the man, determined how old the man would be now, and reminded the client of his current age. Together, the client and therapist also identified ways that the client is able to protect himself now that he was unable to do when he was a child. A few months later, the client noted that he no longer was sleeping with his teddy bear and had placed it at the end of his bed. When asked why, he stated, "I guess I am starting to let go of being a little kid." Such interventions facilitated his ability to distinguish past from present and promoted reassurance of the benefits of being an adult.

For those with a history of interpersonal trauma, it is important that mistrust and fears of the therapy relationship repeating past abusive relationships continue to be directly addressed in the Existing Phase. For example, the therapist may state, "Given how some people in your past have hurt you, it is understandable that, currently, you are more cautious with other people. It will likely take time for me to earn some of your trust." Over time, trust issues within and outside the therapy can be explored, with efforts to discriminate facts based on the present from fears related to the past. One woman frequently would startle and look fearful if the therapist moved too suddenly. More than once, she asked the therapist, "Are you going to hurt me?" The therapist replied, "No, I am not going to hurt you. You are safe and protected. In all the time we have known each other, have I ever physically harmed you?" After the client said no, the therapist said, "Others in your past have hurt you, but I haven't and I won't." An additional, critical, aspect was whether the client was projecting her own impulses to hurt the therapist and this was explored after the client's sense of safety was re-established, with clear statements that the client also would be kept from harming the therapist.

When PTSD symptoms develop in response to the trauma of a psychotic episode, the resulting postpsychotic PTSD can further intensify the individual's tendency to severely restrict his or her experience socially, emotionally, behaviorally, and cognitively. These restrictions reflect efforts to avoid emotionally provoking topics like traumatic memories in order to minimize distress that could foment another psychotic episode. The life experience then becomes one of just existing rather than more fully living. If a person is determined to have postpsychotic PTSD (which can be co-morbid with PTSD from other traumatic events), psycho-education is provided prior to processing and integration. Psycho-education that includes identification of specific warning signs and teaching of specific stress management skills is important for reducing risk of relapse and increasing confidence in the ability to manage stressors. Trauma reminders or "triggers" are identified and ways to manage those are problem-solved. For example, for one woman, a significant and interfering trauma "trigger" was encountering any new person. It is common for those with severe PTSD and those with interpersonal trauma histories who have severe psychosis to have a generalized stress response to people that manifests as significant mistrust/ paranoia that others will harm them. Being able to recognize this generalized stress response and its original source is critical for altering that template of relationships. Additionally, the client benefits from discovering in session that s/he is capable of acknowledging and expressing emotions without getting overwhelmed. The goal is to alleviate enough anxiety for the individual to be able to then explore prior psychotic episodes as potential traumatic experiences and address the person's reactions.

Trauma-related interventions during the Living Phase

Once an individual with severe psychosis has progressed to the Living Phase, to a level at which physiological and emotional arousal is better regulated and there is a greater capacity to examine thoughts and tolerate emotions, s/he is more likely to be psychologically ready to process and integrate traumatic experiences. Specifically related to trauma treatment, Briere and Scott (2006: 74) noted that the individual's status needs to be such that s/he can regulate the "inevitable upsurge of emotion that follows therapeutic exposure to unresolved trauma memories." Further, an individual's level of arousal must be carefully managed during the process of trauma recall in order to be effective (Brewin, 2005). As described throughout this book, pacing is particularly relevant for individuals with psychotic disorders, who often fluctuate in status and in their ability to manage emotionally charged topics. In addition, although the use of projection diminishes in the Living Phase for those with severe psychosis, there tends to be continued reliance on avoidance and denial for coping. Frequently, there remain staunch beliefs and fears that thinking about painful experiences and the associated emotions will lead to being emotionally overwhelmed and, potentially, will lead to psychotic regressions. Avoidance also is one of the three primary features characterizing PTSD. The combined tendency toward avoidance as part of severe psychosis and trauma reactions necessitates patient, gradual introduction of the safety and benefits of processing trauma-relevant material. Consistent with other interventions for those with severe psychosis, then, processing of trauma issues must be carefully paced, with frequent reassurance of safety in the environment and within the therapy relationship and a return to more supportive interventions as warranted.

As part of effective, trauma-sensitive intervention, the adaptive aspect to avoidance can be validated with the traumatized individual: of course a person wants to avoid situations or people that have been harmful to them in the past. If a person physically harmed another in the past, for example, then it is protective after that to want to stay away from that person. However, the important distinction is between actual, immediate threats and memories of a past traumatic event. For example, the therapist might say: "Remembering a time when a person physically hurt you, while potentially upsetting, is not a current threat to your physical safety. The event is over and you are now dealing with the memories, thoughts, and feelings of what happened." Emphasis continues to be placed on directly dealing with memories being more protective and helpful than avoiding memories.

In addition to distinguishing the experience of a traumatic event from recall of it, the therapist also discusses the benefits of direct processing and the disadvantages of continuing to try to avoid the memories. Avoidance of the memories takes considerable energy (akin to the physical effort it takes to hold a water buoy under the water) and generally results in breakthroughs of the affects, thoughts, and memories that are not predictable or under the control of the person (such as intrusive memories and nightmares). Choosing to recall aspects of painful memories returns the control to the person. Also, the more the person tries to avoid the memories, the greater the fear they have of them. Avoidance denies opportunity to see that the memories can be recalled in a managed way and, eventually, integrated into the person's total life experience as one part of the past rather than an ongoing, interfering part of the present. The analogy of watching a scary movie is also helpful: "The first time you see a scary movie, you might be very scared and jumpy. But, as you view it over and over, it loses its intensity over time. It is the same thing with talking about painful memories. Eventually, you will not have the strong physical and emotional responses to these memories or to reminders that you do now."

Highlighting the disadvantages of avoidance and providing a description of the rationale for exposure prepares the client for talking about past painful experiences. The trauma literature describes many different approaches for addressing traumatic memories and trauma responses, including graded exposure and prolonged exposure therapy, emotional processing, cognitive reappraisal of traumatic events, and addressing consequent beliefs and schemas. Graded exposure allows the individual to build the emotional stamina necessary for processing past experiences in a manageable way. Just entering the therapy room is the first challenge to avoidance and this often heightens anxiety for an individual and requires considerable courage to do. Coming to the therapy appointment, therefore, can be acknowledged as an important step in directly addressing concerns. Reassuring the client of his/her choice in what is talked about and changing the subject as necessary provides immediate experience in pacing the processing of topics. As in the Existing Phase, in vivo experiences of directly discussing and addressing more benign daily stressors can be a useful initial introduction to the effectiveness of exposure and processing that highlights the person's ability to manage stressful situations and effectively deal with them. When ready, past traumatic experiences can be broached, with opportunity to see that the individual can manage directly discussing the memories.

As an example of trauma treatment in the Living Phase, a man who was hospitalized due to threatening others with a gun while acutely psychotic, gradually progressed from an inpatient forensic psychiatric unit to a residential rehabilitation program. Over time in therapy, he was able to begin to explore some of the roots of his distrust of others, particularly as it related to severe physical abuse by his father. Education about the potential effects of childhood abuse facilitated his awareness and understanding of his stress reactions and his generalized mistrust within relationships. These discussions were paced to his tolerance, interwoven with discussions of his daily activities, his interests and abilities, and his future plans. The session following his initial disclosure of physical abuse by his father, he entered highly guarded and mistrustful of the therapist. However, when his strengths and ability to survive difficult situations was emphasized and his concerns about disclosing this information were addressed and normalized, he was able to resume exploration. Within this context, he began to display a greater range of affect and increased interactions with others. Despite challenges and some regressions, he eventually was able to be discharged from the hospital and move into the community.

Another male, after a year of therapy in which he had not discussed past life events and stressors, started a therapy session by announcing, "I shot myself in the eye instead of shooting my mother." Although his straightforward comment suggested that he was ready to delve into his past, his subsequent tolerance for exploring his comment was limited. He was able to begin to discuss some of the breaches of physical boundaries by his mother when he was a child, but would become intensely anxious. Therefore, the topic was broached for brief periods initially and counterbalanced with present topics and with continuing to fortify him. The gradual exposure within and across sessions was similar to the processing of traumatic memories for any more fragile client who has been traumatized, particularly those prone to dissociation, with exploration at greater depths as the individual is ready and frequent resurfacing to the present as needed.

With postpsychotic PTSD, processing involves identifying what the traumatic elements of the psychotic episode were for the individual, such as the belief that others wanted to harm the person, specific aspects of a hospitalization, or encounters with law enforcement. Exploring what the psychotic experience was like as well as reviewing warning signs of increased stress and psychotic symptoms bolsters confidence in being able to reduce the risk of future traumatic psychotic episodes.

Skill building continues in the Living Phase, including further developing cognitive coping skills, relaxation strategies, and self-care. For example, identifying facts of current events and distinguishing this from the person's appraisal of the situation and their subsequent responses provides important practice with cognitive coping. Calming strategies are included in each therapy session, particularly after processing of emotionally provoking topics, to assist the client in reducing arousal in session and preparing for coping when the session is completed. For those who have experienced interpersonal traumas, discussion initiated in the Existing Phase of the effect of traumatic experience on current expectations of how others will treat them is continued. Highlighting exceptions to these expectations, both within the therapy relationship as well as in outside relationships, remain part of altering the individual's internal template of self–other relationships.

Trauma treatment in the Living Phase first entails continued education about stress-related responses, about the benefits of directly processing prior traumatic events, and about effective means of coping, as well as in-session experiences of processing and coping. Although reliance on avoidance and continued variability in functioning pose additional challenges to trauma-relevant interventions, processing of traumatic events can be effectively conducted during the Living Phase. This involves working through the reliance on avoidance, discovering the benefits of directly addressing issues and being able to manage the related affect, increasing awareness of the meaning of delusions and hallucinations, and beginning to integrate those previously projected aspects into the individual's internal and life experience. As with any person who experiences trauma responses, reassurance of emotional and physical safety is an essential prerequisite for any trauma work and warrants ongoing attention during interventions of the Living Phase.

Conclusions

The extensive literature documenting the prevalence of interpersonal victimization histories and trauma-related responses in individuals diagnosed with schizophrenia underscores the need for trauma-sensitive assessment and trauma-specific interventions to be part of comprehensive treatment of psychotic disorders. The question is no longer whether trauma is a relevant issue for those with severe psychosis, but how it can most effectively be addressed. As we incorporate the effects of traumatic events into our understanding of the development of many forms of psychosis, we necessitate changes in our treatment approaches. This chapter has described trauma-based interventions across the three phases of severe psychosis to include focusing on establishing safety, normalizing and validating, teaching about the effects of trauma, building coping skills, reducing avoidance, making meaning of delusions and hallucinations, and processing traumatic experiences through graded exposure, with the eventual goal of integrating traumatic aspects into the person's psychological and life experience in a more cohesive, understandable, and manageable way. Integration of these interventions is an important part of optimizing comprehensive care for psychosis.

Chapter 6

Phase-specific group therapies

"Voices are sick people trying to deal with their problems."

Group treatment for psychosis has many potential benefits. In addition to reducing distress and improving coping, participants also can experience increased support and normalization of difficulties, which are inherent advantages of a group modality. Group interventions also provide opportunities to increase comfort with and skills in being with others. Furthermore, group therapies increase availability of treatment to more individuals, better utilize the limited number of therapists trained in working with psychosis, and potentially reduce costs of care. There are some data indicating that group therapy for individuals diagnosed with schizophrenia results in reductions in hopelessness, social phobia and depression, and improves self-esteem, but more research is needed (Lawrence *et al.*, 2006). Ensuring homogeneity of symptom experience in such groups has been recommended to boost efficacy (Barrowclough *et al.*, 2006; Wykes *et al.*, 2008). Variability in functioning, of course, occurs between individuals with psychosis as well as within individuals. Therefore, in order to maximize effectiveness of group therapies, modifications based on the collective level of group functioning also needs to occur. The purpose of this chapter is to describe the application of the SEL model for guiding assignment of individuals to group therapies and for determining the appropriate type of group interventions, based on group level of functioning, to maximize benefits of group treatment.

Challenges of group therapies

One of the common problems in inpatient and outpatient group therapies is that members often vary significantly in functioning, even between those with the same diagnosis. Just as individuals with severe psychosis can be primarily in the Surviving, Existing, or Living Phase, those with other psychological conditions also can vary in their level of functioning. Although those with other diagnoses do not tend to regress to the point of being uncertain of existence, they can vary in level of self-definition, interpersonal awareness, cognitive capacity, emotional awareness, and arousal level. For example, on an inpatient psychiatric unit, an individual with depression may be lying in bed nearly catatonic, be actively suicidal with some reality impairment, or be interacting with others and actively engaging in treatment. Despite observable differences in presentation, often the level of functioning of members participating in any one group in a psychosocial rehabilitation program is too heterogeneous to be effective. Individuals who are reality-oriented and capable of abstract thinking and emotional processing are placed in groups with members who are actively psychotic and have limited awareness of others. This is not only less effective, but often clinically contraindicated, since some participants may progress by directly addressing emotionally laden topics, while other members may become overwhelmed and regress when affect is expressed.

As an example, the facilitator of a general psychotherapy (processing) group was working with certain group members who had the psychological resources indicating readiness for and benefit from having their reliance on avoidance and denial gently challenged. Unfortunately, other members were in earlier phases of functioning and in need of strengthening their defenses (i.e., their means of coping) rather than challenging and replacing them. One such member, who was just moving into the Existing Phase, perceived the facilitator as intrusive, threatening, and relentless because of the approach she was using with other group members. Individual members can become more agitated and paranoid, talk to unseen others, display more distress or illogical speech, or leave the room when the emotional temperature of the group rises beyond the person's tolerance. Such problems are frequently encountered in heterogeneous groups in which some members end up subject to interventions beyond their current psychological capacities.

Another challenge to group therapies is that there exist many protocols for group interventions, but there is a lack of evidence regarding timing of interventions to maximize effectiveness. A variety of group interventions have been developed for individuals diagnosed with schizophrenia, particularly skill-building groups with more stable individuals. Many are stand-alone groups, such as cognitive-behavioral therapy groups and social skills groups. Other groups are part of comprehensive inpatient and outpatient programs. Diverse psychosocial rehabilitation and recovery programs offer innovative multidisciplinary approaches to those with severely impairing psychological problems. Programming for both inpatient and outpatient models tends to target increasing knowledge about different diagnoses, strengthening coping abilities, enhancing life skills, and addressing specific problems, such as substance abuse and trauma. These models have garnered increasing empirical support for efficacy, although no single model has been identified as better than another. Additionally, similar to the research on individual therapy, research is lacking that specifies the phase of schizophrenia or other psychological disorders during which particular group interventions are effective.

Application of the SEL model to group treatment

The SEL model can be utilized in inpatient and outpatient programs in order to reduce these problems of group treatment. Use of the model can hone selection of

Table 6.1 Group assignment checklist

Check all criteria that apply. All criteria met in the lowest category (starting with Surviving) designate category assignment					
Surviving		Existing		Living	
	Severe impairment in reality testing, logical thinking, and judgment		Mild to moderate impairment in reality testing, logical thinking and judgment		Minimal to no impairment in reality testing, logical thinking, and judgment
	Poor attention span (averages 5–10 minutes per task)		Can attend for at least 20–30 minutes		Can attend for up to 50 minutes
	Limited ability to engage in treatment		Low to moderate motivation to address and change problems that led to treatment		Moderate to high motivation to address and change problems that led to treatment
	Limited awareness or appropriate expression of emotions		Emerging awareness of emotions		Increased awareness and appropriate expression of emotions
	Limited awareness of others		Awareness of others/ some interactions with peers		Increased interaction with others
	Limited self-reflection		Emerging self-reflection		Can engage in self-reflection

* If the individual's status, personality issues, or behavior clinically contraindicate group participation (i.e., interferes with their treatment or that of others), an individualized treatment program will be developed.

the type of interventions according to group capabilities and needs and increase homogeneity of functioning within groups. Use of the SEL model also facilitates a common language and conceptualization among disciplines for describing client and group characteristics. Successful implementation requires, first, that all staff members across disciplines that are involved in direct care participate in trainings in the characteristics of each of the phases to ensure consistency. Then, the staff/ treatment team discusses each individual client to reach consensus on his or her appropriate phase assignment. A checklist facilitating appropriate phase assignment for each client is found in Table 6.1. General criteria related to reality orientation and logical thinking, attention span, ability and motivation to engage in treatment, emotional expression, and level of interpersonal relating are used to determine group assignment. The ability to engage in self-reflection is included in the checklist to assist in determining those appropriate for process-oriented groups. If a client displays features of two phases, agreement is made about best fit, balancing efforts to attenuate the person's strengths and 'stretch' capabilities, but not place the client in situations s/he does not yet have the psychological resources to manage.

Table 6.2 Phase-specific group intervention guidelines

Surviving	Existing	Living
Present focus	Present and future focus	Past, present, and future focus
Reality orientation/support/ safety	Psycho-educational/ skill building (basic)	Psycho-education/skill building (advanced)
Activity-based groups	Activity-based/didactic	Didactic/process groups/ relapse prevention
Label and mitigate emotions	Increase awareness and management of emotions	Encourage more emotional expression
Activities of daily living	Basic life skills	Advanced life skills
Basic self-definition work	Basic social skills	Advanced social skills
	Basic cognitive skills	Advanced cognitive skills

**Special issues groups (e.g., for substance abuse, occupational therapy, recreational therapy, psychosis, trauma, etc.) can be offered in Existing and Living groups as basic and advanced topics.

Once phase assignment is complete, groups are designed to target salient issues and capabilities of a particular phase and clients are assigned only to groups designated for their particular phase. An exception is that some groups can combine Existing/Living Phase members together, but Surviving groups need to remain separate due to the greater fragility of individuals in that most acute phase. Groups should remain the same for a rotation of approximately ten weeks (a common length of group treatment protocols), at which time each client is reassessed to determine any needed changes in phase level assignment due to advances or regressions in functioning. Of course, sometimes an individual displays a sudden deterioration that necessitates reassignment of groups prior to the end of a 10-week cycle.

Table 6.2 describes the general goals and guidelines for group interventions for each phase. When the SEL model was implemented in a state psychiatric hospital in the United States, the checklist in Table 6.1 was used by treatment teams as a brief, simplified means for determining assignment of all patients – of diverse diagnoses – to group therapies. Of note, to be in keeping with the treatment philosophy of the program for rehabilitation and recovery and for those national accreditation bodies that evaluated the program, the phases were renamed Rehab I for the Surviving Phase, Rehab II for the Existing Phase, and Recovery for the Living Phase. Use of the SEL model in that hospital system provided a conceptually driven means for more appropriate assignments of individuals to group interventions in an effort to create more homogeneous, phase-sensitive groups. The remainder of this chapter provides descriptions of the types of group interventions in both inpatient and outpatient settings that can be conducted with individuals in each phase.

General group interventions by phase

Group interventions for the Surviving Phase

Similar to individual treatment, Surviving groups target increasing reality orientation, promoting a sense of safety and self-definition, and enhancing basic awareness of thoughts and emotions. The focus primarily is on the present and tasks are brief to fit the shorter attention span of members. Surviving group participants, if they focus on someone outside of themselves, tend to anchor to the group leader, with limited interaction with other members. Members will tend to complete group tasks independently or with group leader assistance, rather than interacting with one another. This process is akin to parallel play in young children before sufficient self–other awareness is developed to begin more interactive experiences. Groups are smaller, generally a maximum of eight members, and – due to limited attention spans – last for a half hour. This time restriction allows enough time to do an introduction, conduct individual mood ratings (described below), and present one specific topic or activity. Each task in group averages five to ten minutes maximum, with the total duration of group being thirty minutes. After introduction of the name and nature of the group and of group members, having each member rate their stress level on a scale at the beginning of each group session is useful for increasing self-monitoring. It also provides opportunity for members to contribute to group in a specified way, encourages awareness of and prosocial responses to the status of others, and informs facilitators of each member's status. A 1 to 10 rating scale of where members perceive their stress level to be at the moment (1 = calm, good; 10 = very upset, stressed, afraid, or angry) is used. Initially, just providing a number rating may feel safer for members, but, over time, members can be encouraged to provide an emotion word that goes with the number. Eventually, the goal is for members to be able to discuss the reason for their rating, although this is less likely to occur in the Surviving groups.

Activities in Surviving groups address the main issues of the acutely psychotic or chronically acutely psychotic individual. Reassurance of safety is particularly important to emphasize, within the group as well as outside of the group. For example, group rules are specified and efforts are made to make the group format predictable in order to enhance a sense of safety. Participants are often asked in initial sessions about the locations, people, and activities that help them feel safer or more comfortable. Activities that promote basic self-definition also are emphasized, including sensory integration activities (exercises that enhance the processing of sensory input from the body and the environment), physical exercise, and focusing on a particular body part and its utility. Basic self-definition activities also involve describing personal physical characteristics as well as personality features, interests, opinions, and hobbies. There is greater emphasis in Surviving groups on how each member is unique rather than similar to others in order to promote differentiation and strengthen the boundary between self and other. Utilization of group leaders from different disciplines helps to address these objectives from a variety of areas of expertise. For example, recreation therapists can develop exercise and leisure activities with Surviving groups and occupational therapists offer effective sensory-integration exercises, reality orientation activities, and activities that facilitate definition of different roles that individual members fulfill.

Fundamentals related to thought and emotion recognition are strengthened through discussion and activities in Surviving Phase groups. For example, the benefits of being aware of thoughts and emotions – particularly to inform about needs and concerns and better protect and care for the self – are highlighted. The difference between thoughts and actions is frequently reiterated and sometimes demonstrated. In general, concepts in the Surviving Phase are better understood if the concept is introduced outside the self first and then internalized. For example, on a board the leader may write the statement, "I think it is a nice day." and then have each participant say the statement out loud. They are then asked to say it silently to themselves several times as an example of an intentional thought. This can also be done with "I am ..." statements to facilitate positive self-statements, first written and then stated. Notably, after being asked to say such a statement silently, one member shook her head and said, "I can't read my mind!" When members express opinions or ideas, these can be labeled as automatic thoughts. For example, one client asked when group would be over and the leader responded, "Oh, you just had a thought about group being over." Given the avoidance and denial of negative affect in the Surviving Phase, examples initially are positive or benign in nature to first teach basic cognitive awareness. For example, in one group, when the statement "I think it is a rotten day" was written on the board, many group members refused to say it. Therefore, thoughts and emotions with a negative valence are introduced in a mitigated way as group sessions progress and as indicated by the overall level of group tolerance.

Labeling emotions, as indicated in Table 6.2, refers to basic emotion identification exercises. That is, different emotions are reviewed, with discussion and activities targeting improved recognition of basic emotions in the self and in others, including the facial expressions, physical experiences, and thoughts that may accompany various feelings. To mitigate emotions is to lessen strong feelings and keep emotions under control within the group. This sometimes requires that the group leader actively and promptly intervene with members to calm them to maintain a manageable "emotional temperature" and sense of safety within the group.

Group interventions for the Existing Phase

Existing Phase groups continue to strengthen self-structure, enhance awareness and interaction with others, and build stress tolerance. Group exercises, for example, can move from the primary focus of the Surviving Phase on self-definition and uniqueness to exploring how members are similar and different from one another, with greater emphasis on either depending on the group's needs and status. In addition, psycho-educational groups in this phase continue the development of basic cognitive, emotional, social, vocational, and life skills. As a bridge between the acute and recovery phases, there is a balance in the Existing Phase interventions between continuing to bolster the individual's coping and self-structure, while also gradually and gently expanding their experience. Continuing to start groups routinely with a 1 to 10 rating scale of perceived stress level in the moment, consistent with the format in Surviving groups, is a useful practice for self-monitoring and sharing one's status with others. In this phase, reasons for a given stress level can be explored and problem-solved.

Cognitive rehabilitation exercises may be beneficial in the Existing Phase, although developing interventions that result in generalization of what is learned remains a challenge. Cognitive training exercises are designed to improve certain cognitive functions, particularly attention, memory, and executive function (Bell *et al.*, 2003). Given that individuals with memory problems have difficulty discriminating errors from correct responses when learning, one promising idea is to emphasize tasks involving errorless learning (O'Carroll *et al.*, 1999; Wykes *et al.*, 1999). Such tasks begin with very simple task requirements to ensure success without mistakes and very gradually and slowly progress in difficulty. Arean (1993) recommended using diverse learning modalities, repetition, mnemonic strategies, and graded task assignments to enhance retention and compensate for cognitive deficits in older adults, and these strategies may be applicable to groups for individuals with severe psychosis. These guidelines are applicable across a range of skills introduced in the Surviving Phase and expanded upon in the Existing Phase, from memory tasks to identifying emotions to conversational skills to relaxation strategies. The introduction of any skill is very basic at first to ensure comprehension and mastery and gradually increases in difficulty.

Basic cognitive work involves continuing to increase awareness of thoughts, such as by having members count their thoughts for a brief, specified period of time. Once the group exhibits the metacognitive ability to recognize personal thoughts, other fundamental cognitive strategies and mindfulness skills can be taught. The ABC model (Ellis, 1962) can be introduced to provide a framework for understanding how perceptions affect reactions to events and, eventually, the model can be utilized as part of explaining how appraisal of psychotic symptoms can affect an individual's responses and level of distress. Specifically, more recent CBT approaches to psychosis have described psychotic symptoms as activating events and work with individuals on reappraising the experience in a way that will result in less distress and more adaptive coping. For example, if an individual responds to hearing a voice by thinking "I have to do what the voice says" s/he is likely to be much more distressed than if the person thinks, "I must be under more stress than usual to be hearing voices." Exercises for learning how to differentiate facts from inferences and perceptions are an essential part of facilitating understanding of the ABC model. For example, members may observe a painting or photograph in group and be asked to describe just the facts about the object before describing their perceptions/opinions. Use of examples based on daily, more benign stressors experienced by group members also can demonstrate application of the ABC model.

Similar to the external focus before internal focus approach in the Surviving Phase groups, imagery skills in Existing groups often need to start with describing the specific details of a designated object observed in a group session before efforts are made to close their eyes and visualize it. Basic social skills can occur, including rudimentary conversation and assertiveness skills. Emotion identification continues and is enhanced by greater emphasis on emotional experience (starting with the physical aspect) as well as adaptive emotional expression, such as fundamental anger and stress management skills. Introductory groups for special topics – such as substance abuse, trauma, psychosis, depression, anxiety, and other psychological disorders – provide psycho-education, facilitate awareness and acknowledgement of the negative effect of such issues for a person, and enhance motivation for change. Psycho-education for groups with psychosis also includes describing the stress-vulnerability model as a context for the development of psychotic experiences. Members identify stressors that may precipitate or intensify psychotic symptoms, delineate personal warning signs of increased stress, and specify actions that reduce vulnerability and improve coping.

Group interventions for the Living Phase

Living Phase groups are for individuals who have a better defined sense of self, more empathy for others, greater reality-based adaptive coping, and a fuller experience affectively, interpersonally, and behaviorally. Individuals functioning well enough to be in the Living Phase, if in treatment, primarily will be in outpatient programs. Participants display metacognition, more interpersonal interactions, and greater stress tolerance. Groups can be more process-oriented although, particularly for those with severe psychosis, continued social deficits, mistrust, and vulnerability to emotional overwhelm necessitate careful titration of emotionally provoking topics in group. In addition, emotional exploration is counterbalanced by in vivo use of coping strategies and psycho-education. For example, at the onset of a group session, members can be asked, "How can you let the group know if you feel uncomfortable during a group session?" Each member can identify a verbal or nonverbal way to indicate discomfort as well as strategies to increase comfort, both independently and through group support. It is important to emphasize ways of coping that do not involve leaving a group session physically or mentally (e.g., by dissociation, intentional distraction, or listening to voices). Across group sessions, members are encouraged to notice increased distress or discomfort in themselves and other group members and to employ their identified strategies. Similarly, although more of the past may be explored, this is balanced with promoting awareness of and adaptive coping with the present and with developing realistic future goals. Advanced topics on self-esteem, interpersonal relationships, anger and stress management, adaptive skills, cognitive strategies, and social and vocational skills, can be offered. Groups in the Living Phase addressing special issues (such as substance abuse and trauma) provide further education, with increased emotional exploration and processing. The stress-vulnerability model can be used to further explore possible factors or experiences that may originally have contributed to members' vulnerability to developing psychosis. Traumatic experiences that may have contributed to the development of psychosis, the meaning of psychotic symptoms, and the trauma of psychotic experiences all may be explored in a group that is safe enough and stable enough to do so. Relapse prevention entails heightened awareness of warning signs of increased stress and honing effective skills for early intervention.

Given the enhanced self–other boundary of individuals in the Living Phase, group experiences move toward fostering cohesion and trust within the group and utilizing each other for support and assistance. This provides additional opportunities to experience positive relationships, to experience greater closeness while maintaining appropriate distinctions between self and other, and to give and receive support and advice.

Conclusions

Group psychotherapy for individuals with psychosis has been receiving increasing attention, with ongoing efforts to boost effectiveness of group interventions. This chapter has described the application of the SEL model for enhancing specificity and efficacy of group treatments by increasing homogeneity of group membership and by tailoring group interventions according to client readiness and capabilities. The goal is to ensure individuals participate in groups with others of a similar level of functioning with interventions that are phase-appropriate. More clinical and empirical work is necessary and important to determine how best to maximize the benefit of group treatment for this population.

Chapter 7

Building the clinician's psychological stamina

Client to Therapist: I have trouble seeing pain in you, so I don't know if you can relate.

The need for building the clinician's stamina

I encountered my first psychotherapy patient diagnosed with schizophrenia during my predoctoral internship (residency) at the State University of New York Upstate Medical Center in Syracuse. When I asked the man – who had had many psychiatric admissions over the years – what had brought him to the hospital, he stated loudly, firmly, and succinctly, "I am here to rebuild my psychological stamina." I never forgot him or what he said, as it instantly made sense to me. He taught me an extensive amount in the brief time I worked with him: about finding the person hidden within and beneath the "symptoms," about pacing the topics explored (I once tried to delve into his childhood and he jumped up, went nose to nose with me and yelled, "I don't want to punch you in the face!"), and about the intellectual intrigue and personal pain a therapist can feel when caring for and about someone tormented by psychosis. From him, I realized that I, too, was going to need to build some psychological stamina in order to be able to work with people who regress into psychosis.

The precarious nature of the individual with severe psychosis necessitates that the therapist possess precise empathic attunement, good clinical judgment, and flexibility in order to be able to time interventions. These requisites might explain why psychodynamic and CBT psychotherapies tend to be more effective when conducted by more experienced therapists. The work also requires that the therapist be willing to explore with the client deep, frightening experiences against which we usually try to defend (McWilliams, 1994). Our thoughts, even our dreams, might be affected (Benedetti, 1987). It requires patience. It requires fortitude. And it requires believing that the individual with severe psychosis can get better.

There are many challenges posed for therapists working with individuals with severe psychosis. These include managing the varied and often intense counter-transference responses that can be elicited, adjusting to the slower pace and more fundamental goals of therapy, and the resultant need to find other means for defining success and experiencing gratification as a therapist. This chapter will describe these issues for the mental health professional and suggest some strategies for building the necessary stamina required to do this work.

Counter-transference reactions

Confusion

When working with an actively psychotic person, the therapist's experience of confusion often is accompanied by a feeling of not knowing what s/he is doing. Obviously, the more disorganized and illogical the client's thought processes, often coupled with rapid speech, the more difficulty the professional has in comprehending the client. This difficulty in understanding what the client is trying to convey, in turn, poses challenges in determining accurate, effective interventions. Further, the more distressed or agitated the person is, the more the clinician can experience that distress, adding to the desire to calm the client, but also interfering with the therapist's own logical thinking. As a result, the clinician often feels at a loss for how to be helpful. Understanding may not come readily, but the therapist's desire and efforts to understand can be expressed. "What you are saying is very important and I am trying to understand. I appreciate your patience in helping me to understand what is going on for you." Finding the meaning in what is being expressed (the meta-communications) as well as determining the most effective means for enhancing the client's sense of safety and reducing distress may take multiple, multidisciplinary efforts as well as time. In essence, it is common for the therapist to experience some of the jumbled thoughts of confusion and illogic that the client is experiencing, and it is important to use that information, in addition to meta-communications in the speech, to enhance empathy and understanding of the client.

Positive, warm reactions

Many have written about the therapist's feelings of love and compassion for the person diagnosed with schizophrenia. These positive responses can result in finding a person with severe psychosis particularly endearing. However, such feelings can develop into a type of infantilization of the client and parentification of the therapist that reinforces regression into child-like states. This is evident in those maternal or paternal counter-transferences that arise, in staff comments about how "sweet" or "cute" the client is, and in efforts to provide for or do things for the client. Any urges by the therapist to do things with or for the client outside of the therapy norm should certainly be examined to ensure that the idea is clinically appropriate rather than a response to the increased parental/caregiver feelings that may be aroused. While therapeutic efforts to provide a safe, trustworthy relationship are important, particularly given that it is often something that differs from the person's past experiences, the balance is in doing so without overnurturing and overtaking. This balance is necessary in order to foster the experience of being a separate individual within a supportive, respectful relationship. The importance of developing this balance in the therapy relationship is highlighted by the fears reflected in the interpretation made by one client about a film he had seen. In discussing the movie, which was about an individual diagnosed with schizophrenia who is befriended by a reporter, the client stated, "His environment (homeless in LA) didn't bother him; what scared him was someone caring about him." Such fears underscore the need to temper positive counter-transferences in order for the client to be able to tolerate the relationship. Therefore, while experiencing affection toward individuals with severe psychosis is frequent and normal, regulating outward expressions of those positive responses is as important as managing other counter-transference responses.

Hostility

The strong positive feelings for a client with severe psychosis that a therapist experiences, while frequently evident and widely acknowledged, can mask the less "acceptable" feelings of hostility and anger that the client is unable to manage and tends to give to others, seen or unseen, through projection and projective identification. When an individual is in the Surviving Phase and experiencing acute psychosis, much of the hostility and aggression is manifested in projections, such as ascribing characteristics of anger, threat, and aggression to real others or to unseen others through persecutory auditory hallucinations. With projections, there is not an effort to make the perceptions fit with reality: the unacceptable experience is projected outside of the self onto something external. Therefore, the therapist is less likely to experience a hostile or aggressive counter-transference during the client's acute psychosis because it does not fit with the therapist's perceptions or experience. However, as the individual moves into the Existing Phase and begins to develop a sense of self and other and more reality-based awareness, transference can intensify. Concurrently, counter-transference experiences also can change. The individual may display more projective identification, a process by which the client unconsciously engenders disowned feelings or urges into another person, making unconscious efforts to have their experiences be consistent with their expectations. That is, there may continue to be some projections without efforts to have them "fit" reality, but the increased reality orientation may prompt tendencies to act in ways that imbue in others the kinds of reactions that perpetuate beliefs about people and the world. This may present in the form of accusations by the client that the therapist has malevolent intent, such as wanting to keep the client at the hospital in an inpatient setting, or preventing them from doing things they want to do in an outpatient setting. Such accusations can, over time, be frustrating for a helping professional who perceives himself to be an advocate who has the individual's best interests in mind and not the untrustworthy enemy the client makes him out to be.

If the therapist also denies hostile or aggressive emotions, within himself and the client, then he colludes in the denial of these unwanted, projected feelings and impulses. Most therapists enter the profession to help others and readily embrace the notion of being the "genuine, warm, and empathic" professional that Rogers (1951) described. However, being able to acknowledge and utilize hostile and aggressive counter-transference responses is essential in the work with psychotic individuals to provide a fully corrective experience in which all emotions are addressed, managed, and safely expressed within a relationship. That is, the therapist recognizing and managing her own hostile or angry responses/impulses – whether stemming more from the client or from the therapist's issues – is an essential step toward the client eventually being able to accept his/her own impulses. Such a process models and contains negative affect and impulses that have been perceived as unacceptable and carefully encourages the client to accept and acknowledge some of this as their own. For example, "I understand that you are frustrated and I notice that I am feeling a bit that way, too. I see that because – as you said – you have been 'betrayed and deceived' all your life, you continue to expect that I am the same way, regardless of what I say or do. So I am just taking a breath for a minute and trying to figure out how I might be able to support and assist you without you assuming that I have negative intentions." Acknowledging and utilizing hostile and aggressive reactions to clients is often novel and uncomfortable for therapists; therefore, supervision and support from colleagues is often beneficial for facilitating this process.

Fear and paranoia

Feeling afraid certainly arises when working with individuals with severe psychosis: from assimilating the terror that the client experiences, from experiencing the fear that arises with the heightened awareness of how bad things can get psychologically, and from grappling with one's own vulnerability to such a psychological state. Additionally, the therapist often finds him or herself taking on aspects of paranoia when working with the paranoid client, feeling "on edge" and more physiologically aroused, scrutinizing what the client says and more carefully choosing words and phrases in response, and feeling an overall hypervigilance in sessions. Effectively working with and connecting with the individual with severe psychosis requires that the therapist is willing to get closer to those most basic, most primitive experiences that typically are defended against, including fears, hostility, and paranoia. Part of building stamina for this work, then, is discovering that one can enter into more of the psychotic realm with a client and be able to reconstitute afterward. That is, you can go in the psychotic pool with the client and find that, not only will you not drown, but you can begin to help pull the individual out of the pool with you. This realization reduces the fear that can accompany this work.

Similar to counter-transferences of hostility, it is easier to feel sympathy, rather than take on the fear, of the individual in the Surviving Phase, whose paranoid projections clearly do not fit with reality, including the reality of the therapist and her intentions. For example, when a client includes the therapist in his beliefs that others want to kill him or are out to get him in some way, it is easier for the therapist to understand that the client is terrified and that these accusations are part of the individual's desperate attempts to cope with perceived threats. However, there are times when the acutely and chronically acute person feels so threatened or the impulses become so overwhelming that s/he is at risk of aggressive acting out. Indeed, if the therapist colludes in denying the presence of anger in the person or in the client's projections of anger, this can contribute to escalations that result in aggression by the client. Validation of the client's feelings in a way that is tolerable, as discussed in Chapter 2, can help to prevent acting out. Also, validating that the individual is able to protect himself may be sufficient to reduce the risk of acting on aggressive impulses. Reduced stimulation from the environment as well as activities found to be effective for calming that particular individual may also be useful. During those times when an individual does threaten violence, the clinician appropriately also may feel fear and needs to make efforts to maintain safety for both of them. If other interventions are unsuccessful, then the additional structure of a more restrictive environment may be needed to help the person manage the intense affect and to ensure safety of himself and others. In such cases, it becomes important for the therapist to utilize his/her own fear response as information about potential risk in the therapy session.

Grief

Given that 5 to 10 percent of individuals diagnosed with schizophrenia will complete suicide (Palmer *et al.*, 2005), the risk of loss of a patient to suicide is great for the mental health professional who works with this population. Those diagnosed with schizophrenia also have a significantly shorter lifespan, with the mean age of death twelve to fifteen years earlier than for the general population (van Os and Kapur, 2009). In addition to suicide and early death, the mental health professional may grieve for the client who does not progress or who worsens over time, for the younger client whose potential is palpable but for whom some windows of opportunity have been lost, and for the older, chronically acute individual whose deterioriation has been accelerated by the iatrogenic effects of treatments meant to help. These issues raise the potential for the clinician to experience sadness and loss, to experience some pain in order to lessen that of another. Also, at times, the clinician finds him or herself experiencing emotions for the client who is not ready to express them. Further, there is sometimes grief and loss as a person improves and leaves treatment as part of progress. These emotional experiences can accumulate in the mental health professional unless acknowledged and addressed as they arise.

The slower pace and modified therapeutic stance

In addition to managing potentially strong counter-transference reactions, the necessary modifications the therapist must make in tempo and approach also pose challenges. For example, it is novel for therapists to define progress as the client being able to tolerate being in the therapy session for increasing amounts of time rather than assuming the client will be able to tolerate a traditional therapy hour from the start. Rebuilding the fundamental aspects of functioning – including knowledge of existence and safety in existence, rebuilding basic self-structure, and establishing basic trust – are primary goals in the Surviving Phase. These goals are essential but require that mental health professionals modify their measurement of success from larger units of measure to smaller ones. In the Existing Phase, there is judicious, gradual introduction of anything emotionally provoking in order to build stress tolerance.

These adjustments in approach are almost always challenges for therapists new to this population, as mental health professionals tend to have trained with populations with greater capacity to engage in the therapy relationship, to introspect and reflect, and tolerate exploration of emotionally provoking material. That is, therapists often are most familiar in working with those in the Living Phase and conducting therapy that focuses on increasing emotional awareness and expression, making connections between the past and present, and introducing cognitive strategies. Being instructed to avoid eliciting and exploring emotions initially is generally a paradigm shift for trainees who begin to work with individuals with severe psychosis. In addition, it is also counterintuitive for a therapist to learn that a more neutral, matter of fact stance facilitates engagement with and safety for the paranoid client while the traditional warm and empathic presentation can intensify paranoia (see Shapiro, 1965, for an excellent description of the paranoid client). The caring, nurturing approach and focus on emotional awareness and expression tend to be what therapists see as their strengths, so to suddenly stop using them can add to the sense of uncertainty and incompetence initially felt. Until measures of success are modified, not seeing therapeutic gains similar to those in the Living Phase can add to a clinician's sense of being ineffectual.

An additional issue pertaining to pace is that individuals often get "stuck" in the Existing Phase, restricting their lives to avoid stress and regression. This can play out in active avoidance and strident efforts to keep things the same. The resultant lack of progress can be quite frustrating for the optimistic therapist who sees the potential for greater quality of life for clients. As discussed throughout this book, it is important to ensure that the pace of therapy is based on the client's ability to cope. However, at times, it is difficult to know whether restricting and maintaining are necessary for the person to avoid regression, or if they underestimate the person's abilities. Systems of care, including treatment agencies and families, can struggle in determining an individual's readiness for new opportunities. Treatment professionals and caregivers can share the client's fears of relapse and, thereby, contribute to the client's beliefs in his/her inability to manage stress related to new experiences. In addition, it is often easier to let clients continue with a routine of activities, such as day habilitation, work, or sitting at home, than to make the efforts to develop new experiences and assist the client in participating in them. In these ways, out of fear or due to treatment inertia, the system inadvertently may reinforce the client in remaining in an Existing Phase.

Furthermore, as discussed throughout the book, the tenuousness in functioning for an individual in the Surviving or Existing Phase requires frequent adjustments in approach by the therapist. The fragility in functioning also means that "mistakes" by clinicians can unintentionally, albeit usually briefly, exacerbate a client's agitation or mistrust. Mental health professionals new to this population are all too aware of this, and often start with trepidation. Being clear about actual intent and promptly apologizing (matter-of-factly) for any misunderstandings often is helpful in mitigating strong responses. In addition, across sessions, it may mean weathering changes in the client from progress to sudden regressions under stress. Sometimes intensifying interventions can help a person to avoid a regression into a more extensive psychosis, but other times added efforts are not sufficient.

For example, a woman who was becoming increasingly paranoid believed that a favorite staff member was changing work shifts to get away from her. The psychiatrist agreed to postpone increasing the patient's antipsychotic medications to allow time for the therapist to work with the woman in testing out her assumption by asking the staff member directly. Not surprisingly, the woman's paranoia diminished significantly after she was able to talk directly with the staff, with the assistance of the therapist. This exemplifies the importance of trying to identify precipitating factors to heightened stress and escalating psychoses to attempt direct, prompt resolutions. Other situations, of course, do not resolve so readily. A man who had been doing well living and working in the community with support through an assertive community treatment program began to become increasingly agitated, paranoid, and threatening within the context of plans for his place of work to change owners. Despite intensive team efforts to intervene, he eventually needed to be hospitalized to stabilize prior to returning to his community apartment. Such fluctuations in status require a shift in therapeutic approach, while still maintaining a calm, predictable, and hopeful presence. That is, the mental health professional tries to alter what s/he does for the regressing client without displaying changes in how the therapist feels. The clinician's potential frustration, disappointment, worry, and other emotions can be processed with colleagues in order to be able to maintain a predictable presence in session.

Attending to the gratification needs of the clinician

It is easier for the clinician to experience gratification and a sense of efficacy when the client verbalizes progress or positive responses to treatment and displays clear gains. Because of the nature of the difficulties in severe psychosis, however, such indications of the therapy being helpful are less likely to occur, particularly during the Surviving Phase. This can be attributed to many factors: the more fundamental progress, limited insight, and the fact that recognition of someone being helpful requires the frightening acknowledgment of some dependence/reliance on another and intimacy. That is, it requires being vulnerable enough to allow someone to matter: a significantly difficult task for those with severe psychosis. For example, during the final session with a man with whom the therapist had worked for many years, the client was having difficulty in saying goodbye and was trying indirectly to think of ways to continue to see the therapist. For example, he suggested that he leave some of his song lyrics with her and then she could return them to him at his new community day program. His anxiety was increasing both about termination as well as how to communicate his experience of the therapy relationship. The therapist's simple commenting in a mitigated fashion, "We've gotten kind of used to each other, huh?" resulted in a significant sigh of relief from him and acknowledgment of the sentiment. For the therapist, this was a considerable understatement of the caring and mutual respect and affection that was in the relationship. However, the gratification came from knowing that this acknowledgment of meaning in a relationship, while diluted, was an important step for the client interpersonally. As another illustration, after several years of therapy, in a final session a woman who had been tormented by relentless persecutory voices for over forty years was asked how she felt about the therapist leaving. She looked at the therapist and said, "Well, you see, I like you being in the room with me" and thanked the therapist at the end of the session before returning to talking with her voices. She was able to emerge from her psychosis and connect with the therapist for a brief period. This final session reflected emerging abilities to trust another, a significant gain reflected in brief moments.

Gratification for the clinician, then, comes far less often from the individual verbalizing or displaying significant gains in a brief time. Similar to the parent's joys over subtle changes in the infant, joy in this type of therapy, particularly when the client is in the Surviving Phase, must derive from more fundamental, discrete changes in the client and the quality of the therapy sessions, such as increased eye contact, remaining longer in the therapy session, and increased conversations. In the Existing and Living Phases, greater gains are evidenced within the therapy relationship in the expanding capacity for introspection and for trust and exhibited outside the therapy by increased independent functioning, work, and social interactions. Working with individuals in the Living Phase can provide more of the typical gratifications a mental health professional receives in therapeutic relationships with clients who have the capacity for greater engagement, reflection and introspection, and emotional processing. Collaborating with those experiencing psychosis for the first time, with the potential for faster recovery and the opportunity to help individuals avoid unnecessary treatments, hospitalizations, and stigma, also can enhance the professional's own sense of agency, efficacy, and hope.

Embracing a recovery-oriented perspective on all forms of psychosis can instill greater hope and gratification in the mental health professional. The majority of the work previously done with those with severe psychosis has been within a medical model that emphasized convincing a person they were sick with a debilitating brain disease and that they needed to comply with authoritative, prescriptive treatment. Treatment was done *to* the client. This model created a demoralizing experience for the client and a discouraging experience for the mental health professional as well. Recovery-oriented practice, with the emphasis on hope for change, empowerment, collaboration, and strengths, provides a much-needed renewal for the professional as well as for the service user.

Working with individuals with severe psychosis can be professionally challenging and emotionally wearing. It is important for clinicians to be aware of this and to allow time to gradually develop the psychological stamina necessary for providing treatment to this population. As part of this process, obtaining supervision is important in order to have regularly scheduled times to "debrief" (i.e., to process difficulties and responses), to receive guidance on appropriate interventions, and to receive support. This is inherent in the training of students and provides an essential mechanism for monitoring and guiding the trainee's work as well as their coping with it on a frequent, predictable basis. For licensed clinicians, even seasoned therapists, who work with this population, obtaining supervision and support is also important. Additionally, a cohesive treatment team can provide support and opportunities for staff to discuss reactions to clients and make meaning and use of those reactions on an ongoing basis. Participating in conferences and organizations dedicated to the care of those with severe psychosis is beneficial. As always, ensuring a balance between clinical work and non-work pleasurable activities is essential, particularly those activities that have relatively quick and more tangible outcomes. In addition, seeing clients who are in the Living Phase, particularly those exhibiting milder problems in response to situational stressors, provides opportunity for brief treatment and a sense of efficacy, to counterbalance the longer term work with those with more severe psychological problems.

Another way to find strength in the work with this population is to utilize the strong counter-transference reactions described earlier to inform case formulation and intervention. This is a basic tenet of psychodynamic therapy and allows the clinician to intellectualize emotional responses to a client in order to enhance conceptualization and guide therapeutic interventions. For example, with a certain client, a therapist noticed herself feeling incompetent, ineffectual, and afraid to say something that might upset the client. She experienced her client as hostile and deprecating and felt devalued and anxious. She was not having this reaction with her other clients and, therefore, believed it to be characteristic of that particular therapy relationship. Once she recognized the ways in which her reactions to the client mirrored his responses when interacting with his father, she was able to better understand his experience. Subsequently, she was able to watch for vacillations in the client's presentation between a dominant, condescending figure and an anxious, doubt-ridden figure. When he was psychologically amenable to it, the therapist explored with the client what was occurring in the therapy and its similarities to other relationships. As in this example, the intense responses to the individual with psychosis can be clinically useful when converted into greater attunement that prompts adjustments in the therapy relationship and interventions. In this way, more difficult counter-transference reactions can be adaptive and gratifying for the clinician.

Conclusions

In conclusion, for the mental health professional who chooses to work with individuals with severe psychosis, there are novel challenges that require additional psychological conditioning. By acknowledging and utilizing counter-transference reactions, modifying traditional expectations and approaches, and utilizing supervision and support, clinicians can enhance their own "psychological stamina" as well as their psychotherapy skills. The successful therapist is able to manage delving into the unsettling aspects of psychosis, contain the intense affect, maintain through slower and/or less typical gains as well as relapses, and sustain hope for progress when the individual (and, often, others) do not. The additional efforts required as a mental health professional working with severe forms of psychosis can reap significant benefit, for there is great satisfaction and reward in earning the trust of the most cautious and distrustful, to be an exception to an entrenched belief that (and usually repeated experience of) "people will harm you if you let them in." Additionally, the greater effort and patience needed to find the person within can deeply enrich the experience of the clinician, including expanding awareness of the range of the human experience, from the depths of psychological despair and torment that can occur to the peak of living life in a full and satisfactory way. Grasping the extremes of psychological experience (in particular, how bad it can get) can foster appreciation of the basic aspects of "healthier" functioning: knowledge of existence, feeling basic safety in existence, and having basic trust in others.

Chapter 8

Conclusions and future directions

"When I used to be unaccepted, I would talk to the air and people would notice. I don't do that anymore, don't need to."

Innovations in our understanding of and care for psychosis are infusing treatment approaches with new confidence and optimism. As a result, individuals who experience psychosis, their families and supports, and those professionals who work with them, increasingly are focusing on fostering resiliency to disruptive psychoses rather than on acceptance and resignation to a chronic, debilitating disease. As highlighted throughout this book, those who experience the most severe forms of psychosis are especially in need of focused, phase-specific interventions provided with positive expectancy for change. The goal of *Surviving, Existing, or Living* was to describe the SEL model as a method for conceptualizing the characteristics of severe psychosis along a continuum and as a tool for selecting treatment interventions based on those characteristics. The distinguishing features of the Surviving, Existing, and Living Phases were delineated, as well as some of the corresponding key interventions for each phase.

A case example

To illustrate application of the model for treatment as an individual advances through the phases, a case example described in the book is further elaborated here. In Chapter 3, a man was described who believed that he had special telepathic powers to communicate in thought with his family, significant others, and important/famous people. His reliance on these delusional beliefs allowed him to feel that he was still in contact with his estranged family; it also served to avoid dealing with the many difficulties, losses, and perceived failures in his life. Individual psychotherapy, using the approaches outlined in this book, was initiated with him through an intensive residential treatment program that was part of a state psychiatric hospital in the United States. He lived in a group home on the campus of the hospital and attended day treatment. At the time that psychotherapy was initiated, he had experienced auditory hallucinations and delusional beliefs for over thirty years. When therapy started, he was still struggling within the Surviving Phase. He spent a significant proportion of his time conversing with and being influenced by voices that he heard. These prominent hallucinations and delusions occupied him and resulted in limited awareness of others. He also was highly mistrustful of others' intentions. In addition, at that time, he only engaged in a minimum of activity each day, given worries that he might miss someone coming to get him, as indicated by voices on his special telepathic line of communication. He had limited awareness of his own thoughts and became quickly distressed and illogical when asked about his mood.

Initially, individual therapy focused on building a greater sense of safety within the therapeutic relationship and increasing the amount of time he was willing to be "in the room" for therapy. As trust within the relationship developed, interventions focused on differentiation, in part by building a realistic sense of self based on his personality, life experiences, and current strengths and interests. Details about his voices and his telepathic line of communication were elicited to begin building a mutual understanding of the development and purposes of these experiences. Fundamental cognitive work included pointing out different thoughts that he had and inquiring about his "own voice" when he quoted others from his special line of communication. Mitigated forms of his emotional experience, particularly related to loss and anger, were introduced and normalized. Other service providers, including his case manager, occupational therapist, nurses, and recreational therapist, worked with him on increasing his involvement in groups and community outings, improving basic self-care, enhancing reality orientation, and identifying and discussing his reality-based interests.

After approximately a year of this type of work, his movement into the Existing Phase was marked by increasing awareness of his thoughts, a willingness to rate his stress level (although he preferred to provide ratings to the hundredths place, such as 5.64), and some limited tolerance for discussing current concerns. He began to express a desire to pursue some of his interests within the community and exhibited more awareness of and interaction with others around him. He had more moments of being in the present and less attentive to his voices and increasing, but fluctuating, trust within the therapy relationship. During therapy in the Existing Phase, he was assisted in building his tolerance and skills for directly and more adaptively coping with the concerns he had been avoiding and denying. Particular attention was also paid to exploring realistic, achievable alternatives to someone picking him up at the hospital as a way to make progress and be discharged from the hospital. The meaning of his hallucinations and communication line continued to be explored with him, as well as past and present family issues. His therapist supported him in his efforts to broaden his focus and his activities, while leaving his special line of communication as an option to attend to or not. His multidisciplinary staff worked closely with him in facilitating outings in the community and directly problem-solving stressors with him as they arose. As he gradually increased his participation in community activities, voices from his "line" remained, but were more often in the background than the foreground for him. This is a frequent experience in which voices become quieter or less salient and influential as the person develops more adaptive alternatives for coping. Some stressful and traumatic life experiences began to be discussed.

Interventions were adjusted to the frequent fluctuations in his status, often within sessions as well as across sessions. For example, he would be able to discuss briefly his feelings about not seeing his family, but sometimes would then lapse into grandiose descriptions of himself as a god. At those times, therapy would focus on fortifying his sense of self and subsequently assist him in managing his feelings of loss, inadequacy, and failure.

Over time, this man was able to directly discuss some of his grief and loss for longer periods, with fewer lapses into characteristics of the Surviving Phase. He began participating in activities outside the hospital with a friend from the community and developing more interests. He eventually was doing well enough to transition from residential treatment on hospital grounds to living in a group home and utilizing community mental health services. As part of expressing affection in a way that he could tolerate, at the end of the final session, the therapist raised her coffee cup to him and said, "Here's to you, John." As he walked out, he turned and looked at the therapist and said, "Thank you. You have helped me a lot." He was beginning to venture into the Living Phase.

Despite the progress he had made, because of increased agitation, the client was returned to the residential program of the state psychiatric hospital approximately six weeks after his discharge. He had remained compliant with his same medication regimen post-discharge, but he did not receive individual therapy, peer support, structured day treatment, regular case management, or other supportive services in his new setting. He was not acutely psychotic, but regressed further into the Existing Phase. His return to the outpatient program of the hospital was, to him, another failure. It was approximately another year of residential services, multidisciplinary treatment, and psychotherapy through the residential program before another opportunity arose for him to leave the hospital and obtain community-based services. This time, he was transferred to an agency that, hopefully, would provide the services he would need to maintain progress. With greater "fortification" and ongoing support, his movement into the Living Phase had greater likelihood of success.

Shortcomings and solutions to treatment for psychosis

This case example demonstrates some of the benefits of conceptualizing within the Surviving, Existing, and Living framework, but it also underscores the significant challenges to progress for chronic, severe forms of psychosis treated with extended hospitalizations under older, medical model systems of care. This example can be quite dismaying for the reader to realize the amount of time and struggle it took for this man to return to the community. However, the case purposefully was chosen because it, concomitantly, highlights the necessity of current efforts to alter our approach to psychosis throughout the world. A critical part of the solution, and a defining feature of contemporary models of treatment, has been to increase efforts to provide early intervention within communities whenever possible. For both first-episode psychosis (FEP) and recurring psychoses that significantly interfere with functioning, intensive efforts to intervene are necessary, including addressing precipitating stressors, fortifying the individual, increasing communication and satisfaction with primary supports, and restoring some predictability in daily activities. The Parachute Project in Sweden is an exemplar of intensive intervention for FEP that includes mobile response teams and crisis homes within the community to assist individuals with psychosis (Cullberg *et al.*, 2002). The TIPS project in Norway utilizes active, mobile response teams within communities to reduce the duration of untreated first-episode psychosis (Johannessen *et al.*, 2001). In Finland, the Open Dialogue Approach to first-episode psychosis has resulted in reductions in psychotic symptoms, hospitalization stays, and use of neuroleptic medication (Seikkula and Olson, 2003). Other countries also have developed early intervention programs, including Canada, Australia, New Zealand, the United States, and across Europe. One can only wonder what the man's life from the above example might have been like if he had received such services during his first-episode psychosis thirty-five years ago.

Such "on-site" approaches to psychosis are particularly important to pursue for early detection, early intervention, and initiation of mental health care to be used as needed over time. Additionally, assisting an individual within their home community eliminates the additional problems of hospitalization, including stressors associated with an abrupt change in residence, in treatment providers, and often in dignity for the person hospitalized. Furthermore, it is an ethical obligation to identify the least-restrictive, minimal risk, effective interventions for both FEP and a recurring psychosis. Therefore, unless immediate safety concerns indicate the need for prompt hospitalization, intensive therapeutic and community interventions are important as a first response to acute, impairing psychotic episodes. There have been significant challenges to modifying current systems of care to be consistent with these concepts, given different health care models and the myriad influences on health care decision-making. Nonetheless, such modifications are critical for improving care for those with psychosis and significant advances toward these objectives have been made in many countries.

The increased training of mental health professionals in the issues and signs of acute psychosis and in effective treatment strategies has augmented early intervention efforts within home communities in many countries. As part of this movement, the SEL model is proffered as a heuristic tool for organizing implementation of the varied, effective interventions currently utilized in the treatment of psychoses: that is, it offers suggestions for "what to do when." In addition, the model offers a potential way for professionals across disciplines to coordinate care. Consensus can be reached about the phase in which a shared client functions, thereby guiding multidisciplinary interventions in a consistent and complementary manner. For example, when staff assess that a client is in the Surviving Phase, they can make intentional efforts to reassure the individual of his/her safety and existence, strengthen awareness of personal strengths and features, and attend to basic needs. Occupational therapy may facilitate reality orientation, self-definition, and sensory interventions for calming the individual. Medication prescribers can collaborate to determine appropriate dosing and types of medications that will maximize functioning and facilitate engagement in other treatments. Without medication, individuals may be too physiologically aroused and emotionally distressed to engage in therapies, but overmedicating also can interfere with energy level, cognitive function, and other aspects important for optimizing functioning and response to other interventions. Treatment by each discipline can be adjusted as changes occur in the psychological status of the client. In this way, different disciplines can complement interventions within a phase-specific framework.

Limitations to the SEL model

A caveat to this book is that it has focused particularly on treatment of severe psychosis as it is currently labeled. It is anticipated that the current definition and even the diagnostic label of schizophrenia will change as our knowledge progresses. Our understanding of psychosis and the different forms it takes has evolved and then sometimes regressed, from viewing psychosis as a purely psychological phenomenon to a purely genetic disease. We are now working toward an integration of the ways in which our experiences, our mind, and our body interact to develop psychotic experiences. This comprehensive perspective humanizes what has been a dehumanizing condition, both because of the frightening psychological and existential regression that can occur as well as because of the dehumanizing perspective and treatment of schizophrenia as purely a biological disease. As part of this integration, we will hopefully come to better explain how those with autism spectrum disorders, major depression, bipolar disorder, posttraumatic stress disorder, dissociative identity disorder, schizophrenia-spectrum disorders, and other diagnoses all can experience psychosis, and discern how these experiences may be similar and ways in which they are different. This may result in more convergent, dimensional approaches to psychosis or better discriminant validity between the diagnoses. New diagnostic categories and labels likely will be produced in response to scientific progress, empathic, clinical understanding, and political pressures. Regardless of where the study of psychosis leads, there will remain those individuals who, at their psychological nadir, regress into a state of existential uncertainty. For this subgroup, there will remain a need for sensitive, specialized interventions in order to help them recover. For those individuals, the effects of severe psychosis can become less interfering and life can become more satisfying, but with residual scars and vulnerabilities.

Potential expansions of the SEL model

As mentioned in Chapter 1, although the SEL model initially was developed for severe psychosis, with its distinguishing feature of significant changes in self-definition, many aspects of the model can be applied to other forms of psychosis. An individual with a less developed psychosis, who does not regress to a point of extreme loss of sense of self, still may display some of the characteristics of the Surviving Phase, but may progress more quickly to the Existing and then the Living Phase. Interventions for any individual who is acutely psychotic need to focus on reducing arousal and distress and increasing the sense of safety in the present. Some ability to think about thinking is necessary to respond to standard cognitive interventions and emotional processing is reserved for those with adequate psychological resources in order to manage the memories and related affects that are explored. Such factors as the level of interference of hallucinations or delusions, of perceived threat, of emotional and interpersonal awareness, and of logical thinking can be assessed for any individual as part of determining psychological readiness for different therapeutic interventions. The anticipation is that matching interventions more closely to the individual's psychological state will facilitate response to treatment and accelerate progress.

Notably, characteristics of a prodromal phase, which is crucial for early intervention, are not included in the SEL model. Increasing attention is being paid to delineating prodromal signs of psychosis to improve early detection and intervention and, therefore, the prodromal phase is an important part of the continuum of psychosis severity. Incorporation of a prodromal phase, including distinguishing features and effective treatment interventions, could be an important expansion of the SEL model. There are some similarities in objectives for the Living Phase and for those at high risk of psychosis. Goals of CBT intervention for those at high risk of psychosis (generally based on exhibiting sub-threshold psychotic symptoms or functional decline in combination with "genetic risk") have included providing psycho-education and normalization and teaching strategies for reducing symptoms and related distress (Addington et al., 2011). In the Living Phase, services target increasing awareness of the relationship between past and current stressors and psychotic symptoms, strengthening coping skills, and developing a balanced, satisfying self-identity and meaningful relationships. Traumatic experiences that may contribute to the development of psychotic experiences also are processed in the Living Phase. It remains to be tested whether individuals in a prodromal phase exhibit characteristics similar to the Living Phase. If substantiated, it may prove useful to conceptualize the person with early signs of psychosis as regressing from the Living Phase toward the Surviving Phase, assessing where the individual falls on the continuum of the SEL model, and determining interventions accordingly.

Future directions

Continued therapeutic efforts and research are warranted to provide effective, comprehensive care across the continuum of functioning. In particular, as highlighted throughout this book, treatment needs to be driven by the immediate status of the client and move away from dichotomous descriptions of the person being psychotic or not psychotic toward dimensional perspectives. The SEL model is offered as one way of promoting a move for both the clinician and the client away from black-and-white thinking to examining and responding to gradations of interference in the person's psychological functioning and quality of life. The mental health field's movement away from dichotomous perspectives on psychosis, in general, and hallucinations and delusions in particular, is a critical advance in conceptualizing, in assessment, and in intervention. Beliefs, for example, are not either true and founded or illogical and delusional. When health care professionals and health care systems maintain a dichotomous view, they inadvertently may contribute to rigidly held beliefs. That is, when the system view results in the options of either a person is right about a belief or she is crazy, an individual understandably may tenaciously maintain that she is reality-based and correct in a belief. Similarly, mental health systems and treating professionals who consider hearing voices to be pathognomic, without consideration of the impact of the experience upon the individual, run risk of the cognitive error of "jumping to conclusions" in the manner it hopes to prevent in the client. Ultimately, the critical measure of whether intervention is warranted for psychotic experiences is the extent to which adhering to a particular belief or having certain perceptual experiences impairs the individual's capacity for daily living and/or distresses them. The more it interferes, the more important it is to intervene.

Conclusions

While research is needed to determine the benefits of this specific model for enhancing treatment efficacy, it is hoped that the emphasis on tailoring interventions based on client status and combining therapeutic forces continues to be a central focus of future clinical endeavors. When there is as much zeal and fervor for learning about the person with severe psychosis as there is for learning about their genes, then we will truly have comprehensive care. When people are truly listening and understanding psychosis, people with psychotic experiences will no longer need to, as quoted at the beginning of the chapter, "talk to the air."

References

Aaltonen, J., Seikkula, J., and Lehtinen, K. (2011). Comprehensive open-dialogue approach I: Developing a comprehensive culture of need-adapted approach in a psychiatric public health catchment area. The Western Lapland Project. *Psychosis*, *3*, 179–91.

Addington, J., Mancuso, E., and Haarmans, M. (2011). Cognitive behaviour therapy and early intervention. In R. Hagen, D. Turkington, T. Berge, and R. W. Grawe (eds), *CBT for Psychosis: A Symptom-Based Approach*. London: Routledge.

Agius, M., Goh, C., Ulhaq, S., and McGorry, P. (2010). The staging model of schizophrenia, and its clinical implications. *Psychiatria Danubina*, *22*(2), 211–20.

Alanen, Y. O. (1997). *Schizophrenia: Its Origins and Need-Adapted Treatment*. London: Karnac Books.

American Psychiatric Association. (1987). *Diagnostic and Statistical Manual of Mental Disorders*. 3rd edn, revised. Washington, DC: Author.

American Psychiatric Association. (2000). *Diagnostic and Statistical Manual of Mental Disorders*. 4th edn, text revision. Washington, DC: Author.

Andreasen, N. (1999). A unitary model of schizophrenia. *Archives of General Psychiatry*, *56*, 781–7.

Arean, P. A. (1993). Cognitive behavioral therapy with older adults. *The Behavior Therapist*, *17*, 236–9.

Arseneault, L., Cannon, M., Fisher, H. L., Polanczyk, G., Moffitt, T. E., and Caspi, A. (2011). Childhood trauma and children's emerging psychotic symptoms: A genetically sensitive longitudinal cohort study. *American Journal of Psychiatry*, *168*, 65–72.

Bachmann, S., Resch, F., and Mundt, C. (2003). Psychological treatment for psychosis: History and overview. *Journal of the American Academy of Psychoanalysis and Dynamic Psychiatry*, *31*, 155–76.

Barrowclough, C., Haddock, G., Lobban, F., Jones, S., Siddle, R., Roberts, C., and Gregg, L. (2006). Group cognitive-behavioral therapy for schizophrenia: Randomised controlled trial. *British Journal of Psychiatry*, *189*, 527–32.

Bebbington, P., Wilkins, S., Jones, P., Foerster, A., Murray, R., Toone, B., et al. (1993). Life events and psychosis: Initial results from the Camberwell Collaborative Psychosis Study. *British Journal of Psychiatry*, *162*, 72–9.

Beck, A. T. (1952). Successful outpatient psychotherapy of a chronic schizophrenic with a delusion based on borrowed guilt. *Psychiatry*, *15*, 305–12.

Beck, A. T., Rector, N. A., Stolar, N., and Grant, P. (2009). *Schizophrenia: Cognitive Theory, Research, and Therapy*. New York: Guilford Press.

Beck, J., and Van der Kolk, B. (1987). Reports of childhood incest and current behavior of chronically hospitalized psychotic women. *American Journal of Psychiatry, 144*, 1474–6.

Bell, M., Bryson, G., and Wexler, B. E. (2003). Cognitive remediation of working memory deficits: Durability of training effects in severely impaired and less severely impaired schizophrenia. *Acta Psychiatrica Scandinavica, 108*(2), 101–9.

Benedetti, G. (1980). Individual psychotherapy of schizophrenia. *Schizophrenia Bulletin, 6*(4), 633–8.

Benedetti, G. (1987). *Psychotherapy of Schizophrenia.* New York: New York University Press.

Benjamin, L. S. (1989). Is chronicity a function of the relationship between the person and the auditory hallucination? *Schizophrenia Bulletin, 15*, 291–310.

Beveridge, A. (1998). Psychology of compulsory detention. *Psychiatric Bulletin, 22*, 115–17.

Bion, W. (1962). *Learning from Experience.* New York: Jason Aronson.

Bleuler, E. (1950). *Dementia Praecox or the Group of Schizophrenias*, tr. J. Zinkin. New York: International Universities Press (original work published 1911).

Brekke, J., Kay, D. D., Lee, K. S., and Green, M. F. (2005). Biosocial pathways to functional outcome in schizophrenia. *Schizophrenia Research, 15*, 213–25.

Brent, B. (2009). Mentalization-based psychodynamic psychotherapy for psychosis. *Journal of Clinical Psychology, 65*(8), 803–14.

Brewin, C. R. (2005). Implications for psychological intervention. In J. J. Vasterling and C. R. Brewin (eds), *Neuropsychology of PTSD: Biological, Cognitive, and Clinical Perspectives* (pp. 271–91). New York: Guilford Press.

Briere, J., and Scott, C. S. (2006). *Principles of Trauma Treatment: A Guide to Symptoms, Evaluation, and Treatment.* Thousand Oaks, CA: Sage Publications.

Calvert, C., Larkin, W., and Jellicoe-Jones, L. (2008). An exploration of the links between trauma and delusional ideation in secure services. *Behavioral and Cognitive Psychotherapy, 36*, 589–604.

Cotter, D., and Pariente, C. M. (2002). Stress and the progression of the developmental hypothesis of schizophrenia. *British Journal of Psychiatry, 181*, 363–5.

Cullberg, J. (2006). The ego, the self, and psychosis. In *Psychoses: An Integrative Perspective* (pp. 42–8). London: Routledge.

Cullberg, J., Levander, S., Holmquist, R., Mattsson, M., and Weiselgren, I. M. (2002). One-year outcome in first episode psychosis patients in the Swedish Parachute project. *Acta Psychiatrica Scandinavica, 106*(4), 276–85.

Davidson, L., and Strauss, J. S. (1992). Sense of self in recovery from severe mental illness. *British Journal of Medical Psychology, 65*, 131–45.

DeBellis, M. D., Hooper, S. R., and Sapia, J. L. (2005). Early trauma exposure and the brain. In J. J. Vasterling and C. R. Brewin, *Neuropsychology of PTSD: Biological, Cognitive, and Clinical Perspectives* (pp. 153–77). New York: Guilford Press.

Dimeff, L., and Linehan, M. (2001). DBT in a nutshell. *The California Psychologist, 34*, 10–13.

Ellason, J., and Ross, C. (1995). Positive and negative symptoms in dissociative disorder and schizophrenia. *Journal of Nervous and Mental Disease, 183*, 236–41.

Ellis, A. (1962). *Reason and Emotion in Psychotherapy.* New York: Lyle Stuart.

Federn, P. (1934). The analysis of psychotics. *International Journal of Psychoanalysis, 15*, 209–14.

Feigenbaum, D. (1936). On projection. *Psychoanalytic Quarterly, 5*, 303–19.

Fenton, W. S. (2000). Evolving perspectives on individual psychotherapy for schizophrenia. *Schizophrenia Bulletin, 26*(1), 47–72.

Ford, J. D. (2005). On finding a mind that has lost itself: Implications of neurobiology and information processing research for cognitive behavior therapy with psychotic disorders. *Clinical Psychology: Science and Practice, 12*(1), 57–64.

Ford, J. D., Courtois, C. A., Steele, K., van der Hart, O., and Nijenhuis, E. R. S. (2005). Treatment of complex posttraumatic self-regulation. *Journal of Traumatic Stress, 18*, 437–47.

Frame, L., and Morrison, A. P. (2001). Causes of PTSD in psychosis. *Archives of General Psychiatry, 58*, 305–6.

Freud, S. (1957). Psychoanalytic notes on an autobiographical account of a case of paranoia. In *The Standard Edition of the Complete Psychological Works of Sigmund Freud* (pp. 1–82), tr. and ed. J. Strachey, vol. 12. London: Hogarth (original work published 1911).

Freud, S. (1962). The loss of reality in neurosis and psychosis. In *The Standard Edition of the Complete Psychological Works of Sigmund Freud* (pp. 181–8), tr. and ed. J. Strachey, vol. 19.London: Hogarth Press (original work published 1924).

Frith, C. D. (1979). Consciousness, information processing, and schizophrenia. *British Journal of Psychiatry, 134*, 225–35.

Frith, C. D. (1992). *The Cognitive Neuropsychology of Schizophrenia.* Hove, UK: Lawrence Erlbaum.

Fromm-Reichmann, F. (1952). Some aspects of psychoanalytic psychotherapy with schizophrenics. In E. B. Brody and F. C. Redlich (eds), *Psychotherapy with Schizophrenics: A Symposium* (pp. 89–111). New York: International Universities Press.

Fuller, P. R. (2009). Surviving, existing, and living: Phase-specific psychotherapy for schizophrenia. Abstracts of the 16th ISPS International Congress, 16–19 June, Copenhagen. *Psychosis: Psychological, Social, and Integrative Approaches, 1*(S1), S25.

Fuller, P. R. (2010). Applications of trauma treatment for schizophrenia. *Journal of Aggression, Maltreatment, and Trauma, 19*, 450–63.

Garety, P., Kuipers, E., Fowler, D., Freeman, D., and Bebbington, P. (2001). A cognitive model of the positive symptoms of psychosis. *Psychological Medicine, 31*, 189–95.

Gilbertson, M. W., Shenton, M. E., Ciszerski, A., Kasai, K., Lasko, N. B., Orr, S. P., et al. (2002). Smaller hippocampal volume predicts pathologic vulnerability to psychological trauma. *Nature Neuroscience, 5*, 1242–7.

Goodman, L. A., Thompson, K. M., Weinfurt, K., Corl, S., Acker, P., Mueser, K. T., et al. (1999). Reliability of reports of violent victimization and PTSD among men and women with SMI. *Journal of Traumatic Stress, 12*, 587–99.

Gray, J. A., Feldon, J., Rawlins, J. N., Hemsley, D. R., and Smith, A. D. (1991). The neuropsychology of schizophrenia. *Behavioral and Brain Sciences, 14*, 1–20.

Hagen, R., Turkington, D., Berge, T., and Grawe, R. (2011). *CBT for Psychosis: A Symptom-Based Approach.* London: Routledge.

Harrison, G., Hopper, K., Cragin, T., Laska, E., Siegel, C., Wanderling, J., et al. (2001). Recovery from psychotic illness: A 15- and 25-year international follow-up study. *British Journal of Psychiatry, 178*, 506–17.

Hayes, S. C., Strosahl, K. D., and Wilson, D. G. (1999). *Acceptance and Commitment Therapy: An Experiential Approach to Behavior Change.* New York: Guilford Press.

Henquet, C., Krabbendam, L., Dautzenberg, J., Jolles, J., and Merckelback, H. (2005). Confusing thoughts and speech: source monitoring and psychosis. *Psychiatry Research, 133*, 57–63.

Hingley, S. M. (2006). Finding meaning within psychosis: The contribution of psychodynamic theory and practice. In J. O. Johannessen, B. V. Martindale, and J. Cullberg (eds), *Evolving Psychosis: Different Stages, Different Treatments* (pp. 200–14). London: Routledge.

Hogarty, G. E. (2002). *Personal Therapy for Schizophrenia and Related Disorders: A Guide to Individualized Treatment.* New York: Guilford Press.

Hugdahl, K., and Calhoun, V. D. (2010). An update on neurocognitive impairment in schizophrenia and depression. *Frontiers in Human Neuroscience, 4*, 4.

Janssen, I., Krabbendam, L., Hanssen, B. M., Vollergh, W., de Graaf, R., and van Os, J. (2004). Childhood abuse as a risk factor for psychotic experiences. *Acta Psychiatrica Scandinavica, 109*, 38–45.

Johannessen, J. O., McGlashan, T. H., Larsen, T. K., et al. (2001). Early detection strategies for untreated first-episode psychosis. *Schizophrenia Research, 51*, 39–46.

Karon, B., and Vandenbos, G. R. (1981). *Psychotherapy of Schizophrenia: The Treatment of Choice.* New York: Jason Aronson.

Kernberg, O. (1995). *Object Relations Theory and Clinical Psychoanalysis.* Northvale, NJ: Jason Aronson.

Kessler, R. C., Chiu, W. T., Demler, O., and Walters, E. E. (2005). Prevalence, severity, and comorbidity of 12-month DSV-IV disorder in the National Comorbidity Survey Replication. *Archives of General Psychiatry, 52*, 1048–60.

Kingdon, D. G., and Turkington, D. (1994). *Cognitive Behavior Therapy of Schizophrenia.* New York: Guilford Press.

Kingdon, D. G., and Turkington, D. (2005). *Cognitive Therapy of Schizophrenia.* New York: Guilford Press.

Kingdon, D. G., Turkington, D., Cullis, J., and Judd, M. (1989). Befriending schemes: Cost-effective community care. *Psychiatric Bulletin, 13*, 350–1.

Klein, M. (1946). Notes on some schizoid mechanisms. *International Journal of Psychoanalysis, 27*, 99–110.

Kluft, R. P. (1987). First-rank symptoms as a diagnostic clue to multiple personality disorder. *American Journal of Psychiatry, 144*(3), 293–8.

Koren, D., Sneidman, L. J., Goldsmith, M., and Harvey, P.D. (2006). Real world cognitive and metacognitive dysfunction in schizophrenia: A new approach for measuring and remediating. *Schizophrenia Bulletin, 32*, 310–26.

Koriat, A., and Goldsmith, M. (1996). Monitoring and control processes in the strategic regulation of memory accuracy. *Psychological Review, 103*, 490–517.

Kuipers, E., Garety, P., Fowler, D., Freeman, D., Dunn, G., and Bebbington, P. (2006). Cognitive, emotional, and social processes in psychosis: Refining cognitive behavioral therapy for persistent positive symptoms. *Schizophrenia Bulletin, 32*, S24–S31.

Laing, R. D. (1960). *The Divided Self: An Existential Study in Sanity and Madness.* Baltimore, MD: Penguin.

Langs, R. J. (1973). *The Technique of Psychoanalytic Psychotherapy,* vol. 1. New York: Jason Aronson.

Lauronen, E., Koskinen, J., Veijola, J., Miettunen, J., Jones, P. B., Fenton, W. S., et al. (2005). Recovery from schizophrenia psychoses within the Northern Finland 1966 birth cohort. *Journal of Clinical Psychiatry, 66*(3), 375–83.

Lawrence, R., Bradshaw, T. J., and Mairs, H. (2006). Group cognitive behavioural therapy for schizophrenia: A systematic review of the literature. *Journal of Psychiatric and Mental Health Nursing, 13*(6), 673–81.

Levine, P. (1997). *Waking the Tiger, Healing Trauma: The Innate Capacity to Transform Overwhelming Experiences.* Berkeley, CA: North Atlantic Books.

Lidz, R. W., and Lidz, T. (1952). Therapeutic considerations arising from the intense symbiotic needs of schizophrenic patients. In E. B. Brody and F. C. Redlich (eds), *Psychotherapy with Schizophrenics: A Symposium* (pp. 168–78). New York: International Universities Press.

Linehan, M. (1993). *Cognitive-Behavioral Treatment of Borderline Personality Disorder*. New York: Guilford Press.

Lotterman, A. (1996). *Specific Techniques for the Psychotherapy of Schizophrenic Patients*. Madison, CT: International Universities Press.

Lysaker, P. H., Buck, K. D., and Hammoud, K. (2007). Psychotherapy and schizophrenia: An analysis of requirements of individual psychotherapy with persons who experience manifestly barren or empty selves. *Psychology and Psychotherapy: Theory, Research, and Practice*, 80, 377–87.

Lysaker, P. H., Buck, K. D., Carcione, A., Procacci, M., Salvatore, G., Nicolo, G., et al. (2011). Addressing metacognitive capacity for self reflection in the psychotherapy for schizophrenia: A conceptual model of the key tasks and processes. *Psychology and Psychotherapy: Theory, Research, and Practice*, 84(1), 58–69.

Lysaker, P. H., Buck, K. D., Taylor, A. C., and Roe, D. (2008). Associations of metacognition and internalized stigma with quantitative assessments of self-experience in narratives with schizophrenia. *Psychiatry Research*, 157, 31–8.

Lysaker, P. H., Glynn, S. M., Wilkness, S. M., and Silverstein, S. M. (2010). Psychotherapy and recovery from schizophrenia: A review of potential applications and need for future study. *Psychological Services*, 7(2), 75–91.

Lysaker, P. H., Meyer, P., Evans, J., Clements, C., and Marks, K. (2001). Childhood sexual trauma and psychosocial functioning in adults with schizophrenia. *Psychiatric Services*, 52, 1485–8.

McGlashan, T. H., Wadeson, H. S., Carpenter, W. T., and Levy, S. T. (1977). Art and recovery style from psychosis. *Journal of Nervous and Mental Disease*, 164(3), 182–90.

McGorry, P. D., Chanen, A., McCarthy, E., van Riel, R., McKenzie, D., and Singh, B. S. (1991). Posttraumatic stress disorder following recent-onset psychosis: An unrecognized postpsychotic syndrome. *Journal of Nervous and Mental Disease*, 79, 253–8.

McWilliams, N. (1994). *Psychoanalytic Diagnosis: Understanding Personality Structure in the Clinical Process*. New York: Guilford Press.

Mahler, M. S., and Furer, M. (1960). Observations on research regarding the 'symbiotic syndrome' of infantile psychosis. *Psychoanalytic Quarterly*, 29, 317–27.

Moskowitz, A. (2011). Schizophrenia, trauma, dissociation, and scientific revolutions. *Journal of Trauma and Dissociation*, 12, 347–57.

Moskowitz, A., Schafer, I., and Dorahy, M. J. (eds) (2008). *Psychosis, Trauma, and Dissociation: Emerging Perspectives on Severe Psychopathology*. Chichester: Wiley-Blackwell.

Mueser, K. T., Essock, S. M., Haines, M., Wolfe, R., and Xie, H. (2004). Posttraumatic stress disorder, supported employment, and outcomes in people with severe mental illness. *CNS Spectrums*, 9, 913–25.

Mueser, K. T., Trumbetta, S. L., Rosenberg, S. D., Vidaver, R., Goodman, L. B., Osher, F. C., et al. (1998). Trauma and posttraumatic stress disorder in severe mental illness. *Journal of Consulting and Clinical Psychology*, 66(3), 493–9.

National Child Traumatic Stress Network and National Center for PTSD. (2007). *Psychological first aid: Field Operations Guide*, 2nd edn. Retrieved Oct. 2008 from http://www.ncptsd.va.gov/ncmain/ncdocs/manuals/nc_manual_psyfirstaid.html.

National Institute of Health and Clinical Excellence. (2009). *Core Interventions in the Treatment and Management of Schizophrenia in Primary and Secondary Care* (update), CG82. London: National Institute of Health and Clinical Excellence.

O'Carroll, R. E. (2000). Cognitive impairment in schizophrenia. *Advances in Psychiatric Treatment*, 6, 161–8.

O'Carroll, R. E., Russell, H. H., Lawrie, S. M., et al. (1999). Errorless learning and the cognitive rehabilitation of memory-impaired schizophrenia patients. *Psychological Medicine, 29*, 105–12.

Ojeda, N., Pena, J., Sanchez, P., Bengoetxea, E., Elizagarate, E., Ezcurra, J., et al. (2012). Efficiency of cognitive rehabilitation with REHACOP in chronic treatment resistant Hispanic patients. *NeuroRehabilitation, 30*(1), 65–74.

Palmer, B. A., Pankratz, V. S., and Bostwick, J. M. (2005). The lifetime risk of suicide in schizophrenia: A reexamination. *Archives of General Psychiatry, 62*(3), 247–53.

PDM Task Force. (2006). *Psychodynamic Diagnostic Manual.* Silver Springs, MD: Alliance of Psychoanalytic Organizations.

Peciccia, M., and Benedetti, G. (1996). The splitting between separate and symbiotic states of the self in the psychodynamics of schizophrenia. *International Forum of Psychoanalysis, 5*, 23–37.

Penn, D. L., and Combs, D. (2000). Modification of affect perception deficits in schizophrenia. *Schizophrenia Research, 46*, 217–29.

Pfammatter, M., Junghan, U. M., and Brenner, H. D. (2006). Efficacy of psychological therapy in schizophrenia: Conclusions from meta-analyses. *Schizophrenia Bulletin, 32*(1), S64–S80.

Pilling, S., Bebbington, P., Kuipers, E., Garety, P., Geddes, J., Orbach, G., et al. (2002). Psychological treatments in schizophrenia: I. Meta-analysis of family interventions and cognitive behavior therapy. *Psychological Medicine, 32*, 763–52.

Pollack, W. S. (1989). Schizophrenia and the self: Contributions of psychoanalytic self-psychology. *Schizophrenia Bulletin, 15*, 311–22.

Read, J., and Fraser, A. (1998). Abuse histories of psychiatric inpatients: To ask or not to ask? *Psychiatric Services, 49*, 355–9.

Read, J., and Ross, C. (2003). Psychological trauma and psychosis. *Journal of American Academy of Psychoanalysis and Dynamic Psychiatry, 31*, 247–68.

Read, J., Agar, K., Argyle, N., and Aderhold, V. (2003). Sexual and physical assault during childhood and adulthood as predictors of hallucinations, delusions, and thought disorder. *Psychology and Psychotherapy: Theory, Research and Practice, 76*, 1–22.

Read, J., Fink, P. J., Rudegeair, T., Felitti, V., and Whitfield, C. L. (2008). Child maltreatment and psychosis: A return to a genuinely integrated bio-psycho-social model. *Clinical Schizophrenia and Related Psychoses, 2*, 235–54.

Read, J., Goodman, L., Morrison, A. P., Ross, C. A., and Aderhold, V. (2004). Childhood trauma, loss, and stress. In J. Read, L. R. Mosher, and R. P. Bentall, *Models of Madness: Psychological, Social, and Biological Approaches to Schizophrenia* (pp. 223–52). London: Routledge.

Resnick, S. G., Bond, G. R., and Mueser, K. T. (2003). Trauma and posttraumatic stress disorder in people with schizophrenia. *Journal of Abnormal Psychology, 112*, 415–23.

Robbins, M. (1993). *Experiences of Schizophrenia: An Integration of the Personal, Scientific, and Therapeutic.* New York: Guilford Press.

Roe, D. (2001). Progressing from patienthood to personhood across the multidimensional outcomes in schizophrenia and related disorders. *Journal of Nervous and Mental Disease, 189*, 691–9.

Roe, D. (2003). A prospective study on the relationship between self-esteem and functioning during the first year after being hospitalized for psychosis. *Journal of Nervous and Mental Disease, 191*, 45–9.

Rogers, C. R. (1951). *Client-Centered Therapy: Its Current Practice, Implications, and Theory.* Boston, MA: Houghton Mifflin.

Ross, C. A., Miller, S. D., Reagor, P., Bjornson, L., Fraser, G. A., and Anderson, G. (1990). Schneiderian symptoms in multiple personality disorder and schizophrenia. *Comprehensive Psychiatry, 31*(2), 111–18.

Rothbaum, B. O., Meadows, E. A., Resick, P., and Foy, D. W. (2000). Cognitive-behavioral therapy. In E. B. Foa, M. K. Keane, and M. J. Friedman (eds), *Effective Treatments for PTSD* (pp. 60–83). New York: Guilford Press.

Sarkar, J., Mezey, G., Cohen, A., Singh, S. P., and Olumoroti, O. (2005). Comorbidity of posttraumatic stress disorder and paranoid schizophrenia: A comparison of offender and non-offender patients. *Journal of Forensic Psychiatry and Psychology, 16*(4), 660–70.

Sass, L. A., and Parnas, J. (2003). Schizophrenia, consciousness, and the self. *Schizophrenia Bulletin, 29*(3), 427–44.

Schafer, I., Aderhold, V., Freyberger, H. J., and Spitzer, C. (2008). Dissociative symptoms in schizophrenia. In A. Moskowitz, I. Schafer, and M. J. Dorahy (eds), *Psychosis, Trauma, and Dissociation: Emerging Perspectives on Severe Psychopathology* (pp. 151–63). Chichester: Wiley-Blackwell.

Searles, H. F. (1965). *Collected Papers on Schizophrenia and Related Subjects.* London: Hogarth Press.

Seedat, S., Stein, M. B., Oosthuizen, P. P., Emsley, R. A., and Stein, D. J. (2003). Linking posttraumatic stress disorder and psychosis: A look at epidemiology, phenomenology, and treatment. *Journal of Nervous and Mental Disease, 191,* 675–81.

Seikkula, J., and Olson, M. (2003). The open dialogue approach to acute psychosis: Its poetics and micropolitics. *Family Process, 42*(3), 403–19.

Seikkula, J., Alakare, B., and Aaltonen, J. (2011). The comprehensive open-dialogue approach: (II) Long-term stability of acute psychiatric outcomes in advanced community care. The Western Lapland Project. *Psychosis, 3,* 192–204.

Semerari, A., Carcione, A., Dimaggio, G., Falcone, M., Nicolo, G., Procaci, M., et al. (2003). How to evaluate metacognitive function in psychotherapy? The metacognition assessment scale and its applications. *Clinical Psychology and Psychotherapy, 10,* 238–61.

Shalev, A. Y., Friedman, M. J., Foa, E. B., and Keane, T. M. (2000). Integration and summary. In E. B. Foa, M. K. Keane, and M. J. Friedman (eds), *Effective Treatments for PTSD* (pp. 359–79). New York: Guilford Press.

Shaner, A., and Eth, S. (1989). Can schizophrenia cause posttraumatic stress disorder? *American Journal of Psychotherapy, 4,* 588–97.

Shapiro, David (1965). *Neurotic Styles.* New York: Basic Books.

Shaw, K., McFarlane, A., Bookless, C., and Air, T. (2002). The aetiology of postpsychotic posttrraumatic stress disorder following a psychotic episode. *Journal of Traumatic Stress, 15,* 39–47.

Silverstein, S. M., Menditto, A., and Stuve, P. (2001). Shaping attention span: An operant condition procedure for improving neurocognitive functioning in schizophrenia. *Schizophrenia Bulletin, 27,* 247–57.

Silverstein, S. M., Spaulding, W. D., and Menditto, A. A. (2006). *Schizophrenia.* Cambridge: Hogrefe & Huber.

Sparrowhawk, I. (2009). Recovering from psychosis: Personal learning, strategies, and experiences. *Psychosis: Psychological, Social, and Integrative Approaches, 1*(1), 73–81.

Spencer, E., Birchwood, M., and McGovern, D. (2001). Management of first-episode psychosis. *Advances in Psychiatric Treatment, 7,* 133–40.

Stern, D. N. (2000). *The Interpersonal World of the Infant.* New York: Basic Books.

Summers, A., and Rosenbaum, B. (in press) Psychodynamic psychotherapy for psychosis. In J. Read and J. Dillon (eds), *Models of Madness*, 2nd edn, *Psychological, Social, and Biological Approaches to Schizophrenia*. London: Routledge.

Teasdale, J. D., Moore, R. G., Hayhurst, H., Pope, M., Williams, S., and Segal, Z. V. (2002). Metacognitive awareness and prevention of relapse in depression: Empirical evidence. *Journal of Consulting and Clinical Psychology, 70*, 275–87.

Thorsen, G. B., Gronnestad, T., and Oxnovad, A. L. (2006). *Family and Multi-Family Work with Psychosis: A Guide for Professionals*. London: Routledge.

Van Os, J., and Kapur, S. (2009). Schizophrenia. *Lancet, 374*, 635–45.

Vasterling, J. J., and Brewin, C. R. (2005). *Neuropsychology of PTSD: Biological, Cognitive, and Clinical Perspectives*. New York: Guilford Press.

World Health Organization. (1994). *International Classification of Diseases*, 10th edn. Geneva: Author.

Wykes, T., Reeder, C., Corner J., et al. (1999). The effects of neurocognitive remediation on executive processing in patients with schizophrenia. *Schizophrenia Bulletin, 25*, 291–307.

Wykes, T., Steel, C., Everitt, B., and Tarrier, N. (2008). Cognitive behavior therapy for schizophrenia: Effect sizes, clinical models, and methodological rigor. *Schizophrenia Bulletin, 34*(3), 523–37.

Young, M., Read, J., Barker-Collo, S., and Harrison, R. (2001). Evaluating and overcoming barriers to taking abuse histories. *Professional Psychology, Research, and Practice, 32*(4), 407–14.

Zubin, J., and Spring, B. (1977). Vulnerability: A new view of schizophrenia. *Journal of Abnormal Psychology, 86*, 103–26.

Index